D1050413

'This book is a handbook of good habits ... Not only medical students but doctors in practice who wish to brush up rusty techniques will benefit from this low-priced and conveniently sized book. Highly recommended.' From reviews of the first edition.

A pocket-sized introduction for all first year clinical students starting clinical training on the wards. It is intended to support you as you meet with your first few patients, providing basic information about how to talk to patients, take a medical history and start clinical examination.

The first edition of this highly successful text was compiled during the development of the introductory course in clinical method at the University of Cambridge. Benefiting from many subsequent years of experience in running this course, the new edition has been carefully planned. Among the many revisions with those first clinical encounters in mind, the text has been simplified to allow easy distinction of basic essential information from more detailed discussion. New clinical terms and issues have been included and the text is further enlivened by many clear and easy to follow illustrations. The authors' advice forms the basis of developing your own style of good problem solving in clinical medicine while maintaining a caring and sensitive approach to patient problems.

Clinical Clerking:
a short introduction to clinical skills

Clinical clerking:
a short introduction to clinical skills

CAROL A. SEYMOUR

Professor of Clinical Biochemistry and Metabolism,
St George's Hospital Medical School, London

and PAUL SIKLOS

Consultant Physician, University of Cambridge Director of Clinical
Studies for West Suffolk Hospital NHS Trust, Bury St Edmunds,
Suffolk

CAMBRIDGE
UNIVERSITY PRESS

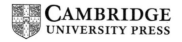

Published by the Press Syndicate of the University of Cambridge
The Pitt Building, Trumpington Street, Cambridge CB2 1RP
40 West 20th Street, New York, NY 10011-4211, USA
10 Stamford Road, Oakleigh, Melbourne 3166, Australia

First Published 1984
Second edition 1994

Printed in Great Britain at Hunter and Foulis, Edinburgh

A catalogue record for this book is available from the British Library

Library of Congress cataloguing in publication data

Seymour, Carol A. (Carol Anne)
Clinical clerking: a short introduction to clinical skills / Carol A. Seymour
and Paul Siklos. – 2nd ed.
    p.   cm.
ISBN 0 521 46235 5 (hardback)
1. Medical history taking – Handbooks, manuals, etc.   2. Physical
diagnosis – Handbooks, manuals, etc.   I. Siklos, Paul.   II. Title.
[DNLM: 1. Medical History Taking – handbooks.   2. Medical Records –
handbooks.   3. Physical Examination – methods – handbooks.   WB 39
S521a 1995]
RC65.S47   1995
616.07′51 – dc20
DNLM/DLC
for Library of Congress   93-46628 CIP

ISBN 0 521 46235 5

Contents

Foreword

The authors call this a 'booklet', but it is little only in size.

Students setting out on the difficult, rewarding journey of learning bedside skills certainly need a guide which is small, meaning 'handy'; at the same time it must not skimp, combining a sound scaffolding of essentials with bricks of detail. The writers base themselves on years of practical experience in their task. Henry Thoreau's 'How vain it is to sit down to write when you have not stood up to live' is cruel advice for many authors, but not so here: these are physicians who have lived what they teach.

My only tiff is with the Introduction where the art of medicine is contrasted for a moment with the science of high-tech diagnostic method. The physician at the bedside can be seen as a model scientist, as Medawar did – gathering good ideas from the history and physical examination and moving on to critical, carefully selected experiments (investigations) for proving or disproving diagnoses. Patients in trouble need good bedside doctors, rather than to be plugged into the high-tech diagnostic work-up bay: humanity, science and elegant economy link up to point the ready way forward.

This booklet paves the right path for doctors-to-be and for their patients – keep it close by you in the years ahead.

Thomas Sherwood
Clinical Dean
University of Cambridge School of Clinical Medicine

Preface

This is the revised edition of a booklet which is intended to be essential reading for medical students at the very beginning of their clinical course. It aims to provide a simple guide to history-taking, clinical examination and case note keeping suitable for the introductory period of the Clinical Course and the first medical and surgical attachments. The booklet is intended to be only a preliminary guide for students, who will eventually build up their own methods of 'clinical clerking' based on their experience, reading, and most importantly, what they see, are taught or learn on the wards.

It is only with constant practice and experience that a thoughtful approach to patients' problems can be developed in association with critical analysis. This will involve a constant effort for students and doctors alike, remembering that the development of clinical skills and the acquisition of knowledge take place throughout a professional career.

Careful and sympathetic methods of history-taking and clinical examination are such essential skills, that this book should also be of use to final year medical students (and possibly to doctors taking higher clinical examinations) who wish to revise their basic clinical knowledge and examination technique.

We are grateful to Dr Richard Page who helped in the preparation of the first edition when he was in the Department of Medicine at the University of Cambridge; to Dr German Berrios of the Department of Psychiatry, University of Cambridge, who contributed the section on psychiatry; and to Philip Ball and Vicki Martin who provided the illustrations.

C.A.S.
P.W.L.S.
1994

Six cardinal questions in clinical clerking

I keep six honest serving men,
(They taught me all I knew);
Their names are What, and Why, and When,
And How, and Where, and Who.

(Rudyard Kipling: *Just-So Stories*, 'The Elephant's Child'.)

Abbreviations

The following is a list of abbreviations used in the booklet. It is not intended to be a comprehensive list of the many accepted abbreviations used in clinical medicine.

AAL	Anterior axillary line
a&w	Alive and well (family history)
AC	Air conduction
ACEI	Angiotensin converting enzyme inhibitor
AF	Atrial fibrillation
AIDS	Acquired immune deficiency syndrome (due to HIV)
AMI	Acute myocardial infarction
AMT	Abbreviated Mental Test (score)
AS	Alimentary system
ASD	Atrial septal defect
BBB	Bundle branch block
BC	Bone conduction
bd	Twice a day (*bis die*)
BNF	British National Formulary
BOR	Bowels open regularly
BP	Blood pressure
bpm	beats per minute
BS	Breath sounds, bowel sounds (where appropriate)
c	With (*cum*)
c/o	Complains of
CAT	Computer assisted tomography
CCF	Congestive cardiac failure
CCU	Cardiac (coronary) care unit
CK–MB	Creatine kinase – MB subfraction
CNS	Central nervous system
CVA	Cerebro-vascular accident
CVS	Cardiovascular system
CXR	Chest X-ray
D and C	Dilatation and curettage
DOB	Date of birth
DU	Duodenal ulcer

DVT	Deep venous thrombosis (usually of leg)
ECG	Electrocardiogram
EOM	External ocular muscles
EtOH	Alcohol
FE	Functional enquiry
FEV_1	Forced expiratory volume in 1 second
FH	Family history (F, father; M, mother; B, brother; S, sister)
FTND	Full term normal delivery
FUO	Fever of unknown (uncertain) origin
FVC	Forced vital capacity
GORD	Gastro-oesophageal reflux disease
GU	Gastric ulcer
GUS	Genito-urinary system
h	Hour
Hb	Haemoglobin
HGV	Heavy goods vehicle (licence)
HIV	Human immunodeficiency virus
HO	Hernial orifices
HPC	History of the present complaint
HRT	Hormone replacement therapy
HS	Heart sounds
IBS	Irritable bowel syndrome
ICS	Intercostal space
im	Intramuscular
IMB	Intermenstrual bleeding
IP	In-patient
ISH	International Society of Hypertension
IUCD	Intra-uterine contraceptive device
iv	Intravenous
JACC	Jaundice, anaemia, cyanosis, clubbing
JVP	Jugular venous pulse (pressure)
LMN	Lower motor neurone
LN	Lymphadenopathy
LOC	Loss of consciousness
LV	Left ventricle
MCL	Mid-clavicular line
MI	Myocardial infarction
min	Minute
MS	Locomotor system
MSU	Mid-stream urine (clean catch)
NSAID	Non-steroidal anti-inflammatory drug
od	Each day (*omne die*)
O/E	On examination

OS	Opening snap
PC	Presenting complaint
PDA	Patent ductus arteriosus
PERLA	Pupils equal, regular, react equally to light and accommodation
PGL	Persistent generalised lymphadenopathy (in HIV disease)
PH	Personal history
PMB	Post-menopausal bleeding
PMH	Past medical history
PMS	Premenstrual syndrome
PN	Percussion note
POMR	Problem orientated medical record
PP	Peripheral pulses
PR	Digital examination of the rectum (*per rectum*)
prn	When required (*pro re nata*)
PU	Peptic ulcer
PUO	Pyrexia of unknown (uncertain) origin
PV	Vaginal examination (*per vaginam*)
q.d.s.	Four times a day (*quater die sumendus*)
RR	Respiratory rate
RS	Respiratory system
RV	Right ventricle
s	Second
SH	Social history
SOB	Shortness of breath
SOL	Space occupying lesion
SR	Systems review
stat.	Immediately and once only
t.d.s.	Three times a day (*ter die sumendus*)
TIA	Transient ischaemic attack
TVF	Tactile vocal fremitus
UMN	Upper motor neurone
UTI	Urinary tract infection
VSD	Ventricular septal defect
WBC	White blood cell count
WHO	World Health Organisation
1/7	One day
1/52	One week
1/12	One month

* For simplicity the female pronoun has not been used in this book and the male pronoun* is intended to indicate that the patient may be either male or female.

I Clinical clerking

1 Introduction

This booklet aims to provide students at the beginning of their clinical course with a scheme for clinical clerking. This has two main aspects:

1. Taking a history and performing a physical examination which is called clinical method.
2. Documenting and recording the information obtained to form the medical record in the patient's case notes.

In addition, clinical clerking begins the process of development of clinical judgment and appraisal which a good clinician has to acquire and which cannot be taught.

The information and advice contained in this booklet should provide a background upon which to build your own personal and individual version of clinical method which will inevitably and importantly evolve throughout the whole of your professional life.

Clinical method is still essential despite the recent emphasis on high technology investigations and computerisation in medicine. Thus, the art of medicine is still every bit as important as the science because:

- Good clinical method is the hallmark of a good medical practitioner. A well established routine (particularly when busy or interrupted) makes it unlikely that important symptoms and signs will be overlooked and allows the practitioner to concentrate on the patient and think about the significance of their symptoms and signs.
- Good, competent clinical method is likely to inspire the patient's confidence.
- Many doctors are working in areas where access to 'high-tech' investigations is restricted for financial or other reasons.
- Use of investigations (high or low 'tech') will be more directed and benefit the patient (cost effective) if they are determined on the basis of findings in the patient's history and examination (or determined by symptoms and signs).

It is for these reasons that at present all qualifying clinical examinations concentrate on the candidate's ability to take a history and perform a physical examination.

The **case notes** form a vital written record of a patient's encounter with the medical profession and good note keeping is essential because:

- The case notes are an essential in documenting the communication between doctors themselves and other health care professionals. This communication is increasingly important as junior doctors' hours become shorter and there is a greater emphasis on 'shift work' in hospitals to cover the 24 h day. Continuity of patient care thus depends greatly on full and accurate documentation of all aspects of a patient's clinical course.
- The information contained in the case notes may be vital evidence in the event of a medico-legal problem.
- The patient has access to his* case notes (in the UK as from 1 November 91) and may request to see their contents.
- The accuracy of the case notes is important for obtaining information for the purposes of audit (a measure of assessing outcome of practice and to determine how well or badly clinicians are performing) and planning; and also to determine what is 'best practice'.
- The information in the case notes (particularly the diagnosis) is used to prepare financial accounts to support the contracting process, which is now the basis of Health Service funding.

To get the most out of your first clinical attachments it is important to clerk in detail as many patients as possible, preferably seeing them soon after their admission to hospital and following their clinical course day by day. Your case notes should include the details of the initial clerking and also the progress notes and should form a valuable reference for revision. Only by seeing many patients in the acute phase of their illness and formulating one's own ideas about them, can any fluency and skill in clerking be acquired. In addition, following their clinical course will give you experience of prognosis, response to treatment and complications that may occur.

No patient should ever be thought of as 'the spleen in bed 3' or 'just a stroke' and the temptation to label patients by physical signs/diagnostic category must be avoided. The problems with which the patient presents should be researched with reference to standard medical texts and by discussion with members of the clinical team who are responsible for the care of your patient. This is the best way to learn clinical medicine, rather than reading a text-book systematically from beginning to end.

Do not forget that illness is usually unpleasant and very often frightening for the patient and his* relatives and that the development of a sensitive and professional approach to the patient is as important as the acquisition of clinical acumen. Therefore, you must appreciate that appearance and dress is very important if only as a mark of respect for your patients. When 300 out-patients were surveyed by questionnaire the majority (with older patients being stricter than younger ones) felt that dress and appearance were important and they preferred their doctors to wear a white coat, be free of political badges and for men to have hair of conventional length. Most would accept more relaxed standards at night and during the weekend.

This booklet is written in two ways that run in parallel.

One gives a list of important symtoms and relevant questions and a simple description of physical signs, which can be used at the very beginning of the clinical course and which should be useful for revising basic clinical method.

The other contains a more detailed analysis of the clinical significance of some of these signs and symptoms. This is not intended to be comprehensive and should be used in conjunction with more comprehensive medical texts as your experience increases.

> At the end of each section is the 'Minimal Statement', the details of which should be recorded even if there are no positive symptoms or physical signs.

There then follows a specimen clinical clerking with an account of how the Problem Orientated Medical Record (POMR) is constructed and a checklist for use while clerking a patient. The booklet ends with a section giving advice to students and doctors undertaking clinical examinations.

Although the booklet deals with clinical method as it applies to adults, the same skills may be used as a basis for dealing with children and the very elderly but with some modification and addition.

2   Scheme for clinical clerking

Patient's personal data (identification)
Admitting details
Date and time
History
Physical examination
Summary of positive findings
Provisional or differential diagnosis
Plan of management
General (or routine) investigations
Special investigations
Progress notes
Information given to patient or relatives
Preliminary discharge note
Final diagnosis
Discharge summary

II The history

1 General

The aim of the history is to obtain and document a complete picture of the patient's present condition which is then interpreted in the light of his* past history, family history, occupation, habits and social circumstances. It may be possible to make a diagnosis based on the information obtained or at least make a list of several possible diagnoses (differential diagnosis) to carry forward to the physical examination for confirmation or rejection. In addition to documenting all positive information, there should be statements about negative data the relevance of which is easier to assess if a differential diagnosis is made after taking the history and before starting the clinical examination.

If the patient is unable to give an adequate or reliable history then the necessary information must be obtained from other sources (that should be stated) such as friends, relatives or ambulance personnel. This is particularly important when the patient is admitted in a coma or following an episode of unconsciousness such as epileptic fit when a description of the event by an eye-witness is of considerable diagnostic value. You should arrange with the admitting doctor to be present when these sources are interviewed.

By convention the history is recorded in the following order:

Basic data (personal details)
Presenting complaint (PC) – 'complains of' (c/o)
History of the presenting complaint (HPC)
Past medical history (PMH)
Family history (FH)
Drugs and allergy history
Personal and social history (PH and SH)
Functional enquiry (FE) or Systems review (SR)
   General
   Cardiovascular system (CVS)
   Respiratory system (RS)
   Alimentary system (AS)
   Genito-urinary system (GUS)

Central nervous system (CNS)
Endocrine system
Locomotor system
Psychiatric/mental health

The history is concerned with **symptoms** which are subjective and which patients will have noted for themselves or recalled after being asked specific questions. The physical examination is concerned with **signs** which are objective and are demonstrated by the examining doctor. For example a patient may have (complain of) pain (a symptom) and you may be able to elicit tenderness (a sign). Some symptoms such as 'swollen leg' will be easily confirmed by examination but others such as 'chest pain' and 'headache' are entirely subjective. It is these subjective symptoms that often require the greatest attention to detail because the diagnosis associated with them (angina, migraine) must be made on the history alone.

The history is very important because:

1. A diagnosis or diagnoses may be made on the basis of the history alone in approximately 85% of patients.

   A precise, single diagnosis is not essential for initial patient management and sometimes there may be a working diagnosis (for investigation) or a number of possible diagnoses (differential diagnosis) but:
   - Patients often like to put a 'name' or label to their condition.
   - The prognosis is much easier to assess when an accurate diagnosis is known and this will provide valuable information about the course of the disorder and how it will affect the patient. This information is important when discussing the implications of the condition with the patient and his* relatives.
   - Information concerning investigation, treatment and prognosis can be obtained from the medical literature if a diagnosis is known.
   - Management is often more effective if a clear diagnosis is known. For example, if untreatable malignancy is discovered then distressing investigations can be avoided and treatment may be directed more towards relieving symptoms.

2. A complete history will enable the clinician to assess the impact of the clinical condition on the patient's daily life, and will therefore enable medical advice to be given with the illness seen in context.

3. The interview may have a therapeutic role in itself since the patient will be in a position to talk about his* worries and fears and you may be able to explain them on the basis of the proposed diagnosis and

planned investigations and thus give reassurance by explanation. One of the commonest criticisms of doctors is that they 'never have time to listen'.

The interview should normally begin by introducing yourself and shaking the patient's hand. A useful introduction is:

'I am (NAME), a student doctor and I have been asked to help look after you while you are in hospital. Do you mind if I ask you some questions about your illness?'

It is useful to ask how the patient is feeling in general and then to ask about personal details and the presenting complaints.

The following is general advice with regard to taking the history:

Establish rapport with and listen to the patient. You will gain his* confidence and be able to accumulate personal and confidential information which may be very helpful in solving his* problems. Try not to spend more time than necessary with your head down writing notes. Eye contact is very important to establish rapport and you will also pick up the non-verbal clues which may accompany the response to a question.

You should start by allowing the patient to talk freely for a time but you should not passively accept irrelevant information. This will be very time-consuming and not very useful unless it is clear that greater rapport will be established by listening for a while. Interruption may be necessary and this should be made in a courteous and constructive way as if summarising the 'story so far'. Leading questions should be avoided but may sometimes be necessary to shorten a prolonged interview.

Although the patient should be allowed to talk freely particularly in the early stages (presenting complaint) the interview should be structured to allow you to record the facts in a logical manner. Facts gleaned early on but 'belonging' to a later stage of the interview should be stored and not asked again. For example the presenting pain may have occurred during his* father's funeral and later asking the patient 'how is your father' during enquiry about the family history will be seen as lack of attention (at the very least).

It is important to make sure that both you and the patient are talking about the same thing. The lay definition of medical words such as constipation, diarrhoea and palpitation may differ from the medical definition. Similarly semi-medical terms such as 'stools', 'wind' and 'water' and also non-medical words such as 'sharp' and 'chronic' (when describing pain) may be interpreted differently and must be defined. In addition there are symptoms such as 'dizziness' and 'indigestion' which have meaning only for the individual patient and always require clarification. English may not be the patient's first language and use should be made of an interpreter (often a relative) if necessary. Otherwise mime or drawings may be helpful. Colloquial English from different parts of the country may be as difficult to follow as a foreign language!

Do not accept uncritically a patient's diagnosis although he* may be correct. For example, migraine is a specific diagnosis but may be used by a patient as a more socially acceptable term for headache. There are also many spurious 'diagnoses' often discussed in the lay press (such as 'allergy') which may be best ignored.

Do not reject anything that a patient says because it sounds too implausible. It may be a 'classic' symptom of which you are unaware, a feature of a previously undocumented condition or a manifestation of psychiatric disorder.

It is worth asking the patient at some stage of the interview what he* thinks is the problem as this may give you some insight into the patient's concerns. For example he* may be worried that he* has a brain tumour because a friend recently died with this diagnosis and his* symptoms are similar. Examination and investigation to exclude this diagnosis and subsequent reassurance may be all that is required.

The history (and examination) is written in note form as concisely as possible using only accepted abbreviations. Some abbreviations are confusing and should be avoided as their interpretation may depend on the context in which they are used. (For example PID means prolapsed intervertebral disc to an orthopaedic surgeon and pelvic inflammatory disease to a gynaecologist). Some of the more commonly used abbreviations are listed at the beginning of this book. When making a formal verbal case presentation (and particularly in the clinical examination setting) the use of abbreviations should be avoided altogether.

2   Basic data (Personal details)

Name
Address
Age
Gender
Ethnic background

Occupation
Date and time of admission
Nature of admission (routine or emergency)
Name of general practitioner

Some of this information will be available from the patient's identification label and need not be asked for specifically.

You should try to refer to the general practitioner by name whenever possible and not simply as 'your GP'. However, many patients like the term 'your own doctor'. It is important to have the name of the patient's general practitioner so that important information may be sent to him* when the patient is discharged from hospital so that continuity of care may be maintained, and in addition it may also be helpful to contact him* to obtain more details of the patient's background.

Ethnic background

In a multiracial society it is often very helpful to have an idea of the patient's ethnic background because races have different cultural and religous views with regard to illness and also there are significant geographical and racial differences in the prevalence of certain disorders. Examples of the latter include the sickle-cell gene which is very prevalent in the Negro population of Central Africa and in their descendants living elsewhere; thalassaemia which affects children who originate from around the Mediterranean Sea; Tay-Sachs disease which is almost entirely confined to Askenazi Jews; and biochemical abnormalities which may profoundly influence the handling of drugs (such as slow acetylator status which is very common in Ethiopians but rare in Japanese).

It is important that the information about ethnic background is not allowed to have pejorative implications and emotional overtones, and the descriptions of 'race' should be as clinical and meaningful as possible.

Example
Mr X, Caucasian, Age 56, baker.
Emergency admission at request of Dr A (general practitioner) to Y ward at 4 p.m. on 12.7.93 under the care of Dr Z (admitting consultant).

---

3 Presenting complaint (c/o)

After you have introduced yourself and gained the patient's confidence, identify up to three major symptoms and their duration by asking:

    1. 'What is the main problem as far as you are concerned?'
or *2. 'What are your main symptoms?'*
or *3. 'What problem has brought you into hospital?'*

Sometimes an initial question such as 'How may I help you?' gets the interview off to a good start and may produce a constructive response.

It is important that the patient's major symptoms are recorded simply in his* own words and not his* or someone else's interpretation of them. This preliminary information is usually written as:

Complains of (c/o)

Symptoms and duration (months/weeks/hours)

For example
1. Shortness of breath on exertion for six months (6/12)
2. Ankle swelling for 1 week (1/52)
3. Chest pain for 1 day (1/7)
(*not* – The patient complains of dyspnoea, oedema and cardiac pain).

Details of the presenting symptoms should be recorded in the next section (HPC). Other major problems may become evident at a later stage of the interview and these should be subsequently added to the list of presenting complaints.

4 History of the presenting complaint (HPC)

The history of the presenting complaint should begin by ascertaining when the patient was last perfectly well and should continue with the details of the presenting symptoms in chronological order.

The onset of symptoms should not be recorded only by date as this may become very confusing and it is usually best to record how long ago an event happened as follows:

6/52 ago	–	SOB on climbing stairs
3/52	–	SOB while walking on the flat
now	–	SOB at rest

Sometimes the actual date of onset of symptoms is useful and this should be recorded in addition to the above.

The onset of a symptom may be linked to a particular event and this should not imply causation. For example a breast lump may have been noted when the breast was subjected to trauma but the lump should not be dismissed as 'a bruise'.

Then follows a detailed description of each symptom, and for this purpose the patient's own words should be used where possible. All symptoms should be described in detail whether they seem relevant or not. For example, if the symptom is pain the following details should be obtained and recorded:

● Site
   Sometimes described but more often demonstrated with hand or fingers. Describe the anatomical site and also the 'size' of the pain with reference to the patient's use of two hands or only one finger to localise the pain.

● Radiation
   The site is usually where the pain is most intense but lesser degrees may be distributed more widely and this is termed radiation. For example, cardiac pain is usually felt in the centre of the chest with radiation (spread) to one or both arms, or to the jaw.

● Severity
   It is very difficult to be objective about severity as pain thresholds differ from person to person and under different circumstances. For example, pain of unknown cause is frightening and seems more intense, and pain occurring at night and when alone seems to be more keenly felt.

   Assess the degree of incapacity caused by the pain by asking questions such as: Does it stop activity? Does it keep the patient awake at night? In a woman who has had children, is it as severe as labour pains?

● Character
   It is very difficult to describe the quality and character of pain but some patients will offer very florid descriptions. In general it is

better to keep to words such as 'stabbing, knife-like, aching, discomfort, colic, gnawing, burning'. The character of pain may be indicated non-verbally by, for example the fist clenched tightly over the sternum (Levine's sign) describing the crushing, squeezing nature of angina.

● Onset

Very abrupt onset suggests rupture of a blood vessel as in subarachnoid haemorrhage or rupture of an abdominal aortic aneurism; or perforation of a viscus as in perforated peptic ulcer. Most pain will gradually increase in intensity.

● Duration

In general, the duration of pain will be overestimated by the patient but should be documented in seconds, minutes or hours as described by him*.

● Frequency

How many time a day or week does the pain occur?

● Periodicity

Does the pain occur reasonably predictably with time? The pain of peptic ulcer tends to occur in the early hours of the morning for several weeks and then remit, only to recur after a further few weeks.

● Precipitating factors

Is there anything that brings on the pain?

For example, exercise or cold wind may precipitate angina.

● Relieving factors

Is there anything which relieves the pain including medication?

● Associated symptoms

Such as nausea, vomiting, faintness, breathlessness. Severe pain of any cause may be associated with vomiting and sweating and these symptoms are not helpful in determining the cause of the pain but help in assessing its severity.

It is courteous and correct to let the patient talk for several minutes first so that you can obtain an idea of the number of problems and then start to define each of the symptoms by careful and sympathetic questions. Sometimes it may not be possible in this way to obtain a clear idea of the patient's problems and more didactic questions may be needed, even to the extent of asking questions which require a direct 'yes' or 'no' in response.

Many patients may need prompting by you asking questions such as:

When were you last well?
What problem first took you to see your doctor?
What was the first thing you noticed?
Do you remember clearly the first occasion you had the pain, headache, dizziness, etc.?
What were you doing at the time?
Have any other symptoms occurred since then and, if so, in what order did they occur?
Have the original symptoms persisted or disappeared and have others taken their place?
What troubles you most at the moment?
Have you noticed anything that makes you (or the symptom) better or worse?
Have you received any treatment? What effect has it had?
What do you think is the cause of all the trouble?
Have you been able to work since the trouble began and, if not, why not?
If I had a magic wand what one symptom or problem would you want me to cure?

It is unrealistic to expect patients to give a succinct and dated account of the development of their symptoms in chronological order, as you will appreciate if ever you have been a patient. You will, therefore, find it necessary to ask a number of questions to prompt and clarify, and to rearrange the story in chronological order.

The History of the Presenting Complaint should include:

1. Details in chronological order of the presenting symptoms.
2. Questions from the Functional Enquiry for the appropriate system.

5   Past medical history (PMH)

Ask:

Have you had any serious illness, operations or accidents in the past?
Have you had time off work or school because of illness?

*Have you had rheumatic fever, severe measles, whooping
    cough, scarlet fever, diabetes, jaundice or tuberculosis?
Have you had medical examinations for employment or
    insurance purposes and what was the result?
Do you have children (women) and were there any problems
    during the pregnancy or labour?*

The past medical history should include an account of all previous
illnesses or operations, whether apparently important or not. The
patient is first given the opportunity to recall past illnesses and then
certain events enquired for specifically.

If the patient has had illnesses or operations in the past, note the date
and whether recovery was uncomplicated and complete. Some idea of
the severity of the illness or operation may be gained by asking how
long the patient was in hospital, in bed and/or away from work. In
'doubtful' cases do not uncritically accept the 'diagnosis' that the
patient gives you, but ask him* to describe the illness and form your
own conclusion. An alternative is to ask the patient who it was that
made the diagnosis and on what basis. It is often helpful to enquire
whether the patient has ever had a general medical examination in the
past for insurance or employment purposes, and if so, whether he* was
pronounced fit. If he* was in the Armed Forces, ask whether he* was
discharged A1.

If you have access to the hospital case notes, the past medical history
can be verified and further details obtained. All past complaints should
be recorded in chronological order using either the age of the patient at
the time or the year in which the event occurred.

Ask specifically about:

● Serious medical illness

Rheumatic fever was sometimes called 'growing pains'. Perhaps the
    patient was confined to bed for several months, not allowed to do
    games at school, or told of a heart murmur. The main symptom
    which is likely to be remembered is joint pain severe enough to
    have had the limbs wrapped in cotton wool. The long-term effects
    of rheumatic fever are on the heart, causing valvular heart disease
    (particularly mitral stenosis).

Severe measles and whooping cough may lead to chronic lung
    disease, particularly bronchiectasis.

Scarlet fever may cause chronic kidney disease.

The history of tuberculosis should be documented in detail,
    particularly with regard to treatment. There were many

mutilating operations performed prior to the mid-1950s, the complications of which are now becoming apparent. There may be a reactivation of tuberculosis unless the patient received a full course of antibiotics, and this information should be sought.

- Surgical illness or operations
  Note operative details, complications and extent of recovery, including post-operative medication.

- Accidents
  Did these occur by chance or were they related to occupation? There may be the possibility of litigation associated with the latter and symptoms may be exaggerated to improve the chance of winning compensation.

- Pregnancies
  Document the number of live and dead births and complications of the pregnancy and delivery particularly raised blood pressure and haemorrhage.
  Written para $2+^0$ – where main number is live births and suffix indicates dead births. FTND is the accepted abbreviation for full term normal delivery.

6   Family history (FH)

Ask:

Are there any medical conditions such as diabetes, thyroid disease, raised blood pressure, heart attacks, strokes or asthma that tend to run in your family?
How old was your father/mother when he/she died and do you know the cause of death?
How many brothers/sisters do you have and how are they?
How many children do you have? How old are they and are they keeping well?

The purpose of taking a family history is to obtain evidence of similar disease in other members of the family in order to help in the patient's diagnosis and also to be able to give advice to other members of the family. Some diseases are clearly inherited in Mendelian fashion whereas in others it may be a susceptibility that appears to be inherited. Clustering of disease in a family may indicate the same causal agent.

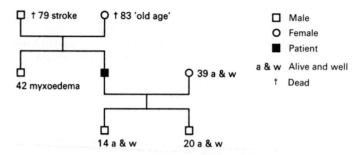

Fig. 1. Family history.

Document whether there are any illnesses that run in the family asking particularly about diabetes, thyroid disease, heart disease, hypertension, peptic ulcers and atopy (hayfever, eczema or asthma). Record the state of health of all immediate relatives and, if any such relative has died, state at what age and ascertain the cause as tactfully as possible.

These data may be recorded either as a family tree (see Fig. 1) or as follows:

Father	†79	stroke
Mother	†83	'old age'
1 Brother	42	myxoedema
Wife	39	a&w
2 Sons	14	a&w
	20	a&w

No hypertension, premature vascular disease, diabetes, thyroid disease, asthma.

a&w = alive and well
  † = dead

7   Medication and allergy history

Ask:

Are you taking any medicines, pills or tablets?
If so, what are they, how long have you been taking them and
  for what condition?

Medication

Document exactly what treatment the patient is taking and its duration and whether other treatments have been discontinued recently. Many medical problems (particularly in the elderly) are caused by side effects of medication (iatrogenic disease). If possible look at the medicine bottles and identify the medication. Many patients now have a computerised list of their medication from their general practitioner.

Ask whether the patient is taking any medication which is not prescribed. This may be purchased over the counter or be a 'recreational drug'.

Women may omit to mention taking an oral contraceptive pill ('the pill') or HRT and these questions should be asked specifically.

Document the medication as follows:

Digoxin 250 μg od for 5 years
Amoxycillin 250 mg t.d.s. for the last 4/7
Finished a 5/7 course of ofloxacin 4/7 ago

Ask:

Do you have any allergies?
Do you have hayfever, eczema or asthma?
Have you ever had any reaction to a medicine, tablet or food?

Allergy

Establish that these are true allergies because there are many non-specific symptoms and illnesses that are often attributed to 'allergy'. It is very important to establish correctly a diagnosis of penicillin hypersensitivity because further exposure could cause a severe reaction. However, if the diagnosis is not certain then the patient may be denied a life-saving treatment. True penicillin hypersensitivity causes a reaction that varies from urticaria and wheezing to anaphylaxis and circulatory collapse. Many other non-specific symptoms may be attributed to penicillin treatment and can be ignored. A skin reaction that is usually not repeated occurs when ampicillin is used to treat a viral infection and this must be distinguished from true hypersensitivity.

8   Personal and social history (PH and SH)

Ask:

How much alcohol do you drink?
Do you smoke? If so, how much? and what?/If not, have you
*   ever? and when did you stop?*
Who is with you at home?
How do you manage at home?
Do you have pets at home or live near farmland?
Have you been abroad in the last 2 years?
Do you go out to work? If so what is your job?
Is driving a part of your job and, if so, do you have an HGV or
*   PSV licence?*

The personal and social history should provide a picture of the patient's background, occupation, home environment, worries, personality, and alcohol and tobacco consumption. Much of this may have already been established during the course of the history but, if not, further specific details should be sought. The amount of detail required will vary a great deal depending on the likely diagnosis of the illness and the suspected environmental situation.

Alcohol consumption

Document the number of units of alcohol consumed in a week. One unit is approximately 8 gm of pure alcohol and is contained in half-a-pint of beer, a 'pub-measure' of spirits, a glass of wine or a glass of fortified wine (sherry, port). The alcohol content of beer and wine varies so this is only an approximation. Most alcoholic drinks give an indication of their alcohol content, usually by stating the volume/ volume percentage. Establish the pattern of drinking – whether daily intake or in 'binges'.

The recommended maximum weekly 'safe' intake for a man is 21 units and for a woman is 14 units, but it is unlikely that clinically significant alcohol-related problems will be encountered until a patient is drinking in excess of 50 units a week. A patient will tend to underestimate his* consumption of alcohol, particularly if it is excessive, and patients who have a drinking problem may be identified using the 'CAGE' questions as follows:

1. Have you ever felt that you should **C**ut down on your drinking?
2. Have people **A**nnoyed you by criticising your drinking?
3. Have you ever felt **G**uilty about your drinking?

4. Have you ever had a drink first thing in the morning to steady your nerves or get rid of a hangover (Eye-opener)?

Alcohol dependence is likely if the patient gives two or more positive answers. Additional pointers may include unstable work and marital history and certain high risk occupations (such as publican and doctor). Symptoms include morning headache, nausea and vomiting and evasive answers to questions about alcohol.

Tobacco consumption

Ask about the number of cigarettes smoked per day. An 'auction' may be necessary where the patient starts with a small number and you suggest a larger one until a compromise is reached. Some people (particularly in USA) will measure their tobacco consumption in terms of 'packs per week' where a 'pack' is 20 cigarettes.

For pipe smokers and those who roll their own cigarettes the number of ounces of tobacco a week is usually easy to establish. One ounce of tobacco is the approximate equivalent of 30 cigarettes and the use of more than three ounces of tobacco a week identifies a 'heavy smoker'. Tobacco is now sold as pouches of 25 gm and this is the approximate equivalent of one ounce. Most patients (particularly in UK) still talk of 'ounces' of tobacco. If a patient says that he* does not smoke, ask if he* ever has done so (he* may have given up a few days before). Remember that 'smoking' to some people means using marijuana (cannabis, hemp, grass, pot).

The risk of developing lung cancer remains for at least 15 years after smoking has been discontinued and it is not known whether an ex-smoker ever achieves the risk of a life-long non-smoker in terms of cardiovascular risk. Smoking also causes chronic bronchitis and contributes to mouth and bladder cancer. Pipe smokers have a lower risk of lung disease and cancer as do cigar smokers unless they have changed from cigarettes to cigars.

There is increasing evidence that passive smoking contributes to lung cancer and ischaemic heart disease in adults and to lung disease in the children of smokers. It may be appropriate to ask about the working or social environment with regard to exposure to cigarette smoke.

Present and past occupations

Note particularly, the nature of the job and whether there is, or was, any occupational hazard such as exposure to dusts or chemicals, particularly asbestos. Establish what the patient actually does during his* work as it may be physically demanding, involve climbing ladders and so on. The job may be causing or contributing to the illness and the illness may have a profound effect on the ability to perform the job.

Driving may pose a particular problem because, at the very least, people value the independence that it affords (particularly in the country) and at the worst, the patient's job may depend on being able to drive. There are many medical conditions that may make driving hazardous and these include poor eyesight, sudden disabling attacks of giddiness or loss of consciousness (particularly epilepsy) and, most commonly, heart disease. The criteria for establishing fitness to drive on medical grounds are much more stringent for vocational licences such as Heavy Goods Vehicle (HGV), and patients whose livelihoods depend upon these licences may not disclose symptoms which may lead to their withdrawal. The implications of diagnoses such as epilepsy or angina will tend to be greater for people who depend upon driving for their livelihood and perhaps the criteria for making these diagnoses should be considered particularly carefully.

Some spouses will object to the assumption that they do not 'work'. It is better to ask women if they 'go out to work', or work from the home (in addition to housework!).

Enforced unemployment has many implications that are not only social but may contribute to ill health. If a person is not in regular employment ask why, and what steps are being taken to find a job. If it is a medical condition that is preventing him* from working then this needs to be relieved, and if this is not possible then help should be sought from the various social agencies in order to find suitable employment.

People who are self-employed tend to persist with their job for as long as possible and although they want to be fit they are often unable or unwilling to take the time off work that is necessary for investigations (time is money).

Circumstances and conditions at home

These may be relevant to the patient's admission and are very relevant to the patient's discharge from hospital. For example, it is important to establish whether an elderly and frail person has stairs to climb to the bedroom or toilet facilities, or perhaps there is an outside toilet. Patients may require a 'home visit' prior to discharge from hospital, when they visit their home for a few hours with an occupational therapist and physiotherapist who are able to assess the patient's home needs in relation to his* illness or disability.

Mention should also be made of any pets, such as dogs, budgerigars, parrots or pigeons since these animals may cause disease or be the carriers of infective organisms. Human disease acquired from animals is termed zoonosis.

Recent travel abroad

Note countries visited, and whether vaccinations were performed before leaving the home country and whether prophylaxis (against malaria for example) was continued on return.

Further information

When indicated, further information such as education, domestic and financial worries or sexual history may be helpful. In addition, knowledge of salt intake (in hypertension), caffeine consumption (palpitation) and diet (obesity or hypercholesterolaemia) may be appropriate.

9 Minimal statement of personal and social history

> No medication
> No allergies
> Smokes 25 cigarettes per day
> Alcohol socially < 6 units/week
> Baker for 30 years – flour dust + +
> Lives with wife and two sons in their own home
> No social or financial problems

III Psychiatric history

1 Complaints

List the patient's presenting complaints, verbatim if possible.

2 History of the presenting complaint

Obtain a detailed account of the illness from the earliest time that a change was noted. The sequence of the various symptoms should be dated approximately, and a record made of changes in the patient's life situation as a result of the illness, and his* reactions to them (e.g. sick leave or loss of job, limitation of social activities, estrangement from spouse, conflict with the law). Note the reason for, and mode of, admission to hospital. Do not limit yourself to a mere statement of the patient's spontaneous complaints. You should enquire about other important symptoms, especially presence or absence of other psychological symptoms.

For example, a complaint of 'depression' should always be followed by questions about the quality of the mood change and any variation, concentration, interest, energy, sleep, appetite, guilt, self-pity, etc.

3 Previous history

- *Psychiatric*
  Note any previous nervous or mental illness; whether or not in circumscribed attacks; whether treated, and if so, where.

- *Medical (See p. 13.)*

4 Family history

- *Parents*
  Age, occupation, health and personality.
  If deceased, age at death and cause.
  Note patient's age at death of parent.

- *Sibs*
  List in chronological order by age, marital state, occupation,
  health and personality.
  Record the presence of any nervous or mental trouble,
  including excess alcohol consumption.

- *Early home environment*
  Enquire about the environment in which the patient spent his*
  childhood (e.g. whether brought up by parents or others),
  home atmosphere, relations between parents and between
  parents and children, financial state of family and material
  environment.

5 Personal history

- *Date and place of birth*
  Full term or premature, normal delivery or otherwise, birth
  injuries.

- *Health during childhood*
  Delicate or healthy, childhood illnesses.

- *Neurotic traits*
  Excessive 'nervousness' or shyness, also enuresis, food fads,
  temper tantrums, sleep-walking.

- *School record*
  School leaving age, names and types of schools attended and
  academic progress, success in making friends, ability to relate
  to teachers, participation in games, homesickness (where
  appropriate), disciplinary difficulties, bullying, school phobia
  (particularly after the age of 10 yr).

● *Work record*
  List in chronological order, jobs held, with reasons for taking and leaving them. Also, note any service in the Armed Forces and rank attained.

● *Marital history*
  Age at marriage, duration of acquaintance before marriage and of engagement. Spouse's age, occupation and personality. Compatibility, sharing of responsibilities. Sexual difficulties, contraceptive measures. List of children with names and ages, and brief note of health and personality of each.

● *Sexual adjustment*
  Age at onset of puberty (menarche, voice-breaking) and how these changes were regarded. In female patients, regularity of periods, and presence of pain or emotional disturbance before or during them, also age at menopause and any accompanying physical or psychological disturbance.

The following topics are often embarrassing to patients and if not immediately relevant may be omitted. However, if there is any evidence of sexual difficulty or unusual sexual interest, these areas will have to be explored:

  Knowledge of the facts of life and how acquired.
  Masturbation, associated fantasies and attitudes towards them.
  Homosexual feelings during adolescence or later.
  Traumatic sexual experiences during childhood (sexual abuse).

● *Present home situation*
  Attitude to housing, financial and social circumstances. Problems in family relationships and recent stresses within and outside the home.

● *Personality before illness*
  The personal history may indicate stability, permanency, ability to accept responsibility and whether the patient is positive and effective, or negative and inadequate. Also, how far the present state contrasts with his previous personality.*

● *Social relations*
  Attitudes towards relatives and friends, ability to mix easily. Attitudes towards authority (including anti-social trends,

stealing, lying, etc.), towards religion and politics. Record
any group activities in clubs, societies, etc. How is leisure
spent? Hobbies and interests, social aspirations.

● Mood
Whether habitually cheerful or despondent, anxious or placid,
optimistic or pessimistic, warm-hearted or emotionally cold.
Ask particularly, whether mood is relatively stable or prone to
fluctuations, regular or irregular, and whether predictable or
not.

● Character
Self-confident, or shy and timid. Self-reliant in planning and
judgment, or dependent on others; enterprising, or preferring
the old familiar. Ask particularly whether patient is
scrupulous, conscientious, prone to set himself* high
standards, punctual and methodical, or capricious,
unreliable, impulsive. (Strictness, fussiness and rigid
adherence to routine are often associated with extreme
conscientiousness.)

● Activity
Whether active and energetic, or sluggish and easily fatigued.
Whether energy output is sustained or fitful.

● Habits
Food fads, excretory function, alcohol, tobacco, drugs.
Concern over health, frequent taking of patent medicines.

● Sleep
Quality, quantity, any recent changes, snoring, waking
irritabililty, anxiety or headache, nightmares, sleep paralysis,
hallucinatory experiences.

6   Mental state at inverview

● Appearance and behaviour
Tidy or ill-kempt, calm, tense or agitated, cheerful or glum, easy
or difficult to make contact with. Any noticeable oddities
such as mannerisms or gestures.

- Mood
    Appearance gives some indication of this. Non-committal
    questions should be asked: 'How do you feel in yourself?';
    'How are your spirits?'. Many varieties of mood may be
    present – not merely degrees of happiness or sadness, but
    irritability, fear, worry, bewilderment, apathy. Note how
    constant the mood is, whether the patient seems capable of
    'snapping out of it' temporarily, and how far the mood is
    appropriate to the circumstances. Suicidal ideation and
    plans.

- Talk
    Form rather than content is considered here.
    Does the patient talk readily or reluctantly, at normal speed or
        very fast or very slowly, to the point or discursively, is the
        patient coherent, any strange words or puns, any sudden
        stops or changes in topic.
    Give verbatim examples (where appropriate).

- Thought content
    (i) Preoccupations and fears of ill-health, insanity, poverty,
        guilt, etc.
        Any obsessive–compulsive phenomena, such as thoughts or
        impulses repeatedly intruding against the patient's will?
        Does he* have to repeat actions unnecessarily?
        Does he* realise how illogical they are?
        Phobias – specific and social.
    (ii) Delusions and misinterpretations
        Does the patient show abnormal attitudes towards people or
        things?
        Is he* treated well or in some special way by people around
        him*?
        Are people talking about him* or looking at him*?
        Does he feel under any influence or control?
        Has he* had perplexing experiences?
        Does he* read in the newspapers, see on TV or hear on the
        radio, things referring specifically to him*?
        Does he* deprecate and blame himself* (for example in his*
        morals, character, health or possessions) or does he* seem
        to regard himself* in an inflated and grandiose way?
        Give verbatim examples (where appropriate).

(iii) *Disorders of perception*
Does he* see things?
Do his* thoughts turn to words in his* head?
Does he* hear voices giving him orders or criticising him or interfering with his* thoughts?
Does he* experience peculiar bodily sensation, vibrations or electricity etc.?
Note the frequency, vividness and timing of hallucinations, as well as the patient's reaction to them and beliefs about their origin.
Give verbatim examples (where appropriate).

7 Intellectual function

Assessed as described in the section on neurological examination (chapter 6.2).

Delusions are beliefs often of a persecutory and bizarre nature that are held despite rational contradiction. Patients may believe that they are controlled by psychic or physical forces, such as electricity or radiowaves, and believe that people are inserting thoughts into their minds.

Hallucinations are perceptions in the absence of appropriate stimuli and may be auditory, visual or olfactory. The 'voices' that a patient hears typically come from outside their head and may talk to them in the second person (e.g. 'You are being followed'), or discuss them in the third person often in hostile terms (e.g. 'He is a pervert and we are going to kill him').

Schizophrenia is a chronic relapsing psychotic illness presenting with acute symptoms that may progress to chronic symptoms leading to disintegration of personality and gross impairment of social functioning.

The presenting symptoms may be divided into:
- Acute positive symptoms, such as hallucinations (particularly auditory), thought disorder (loosening of associations), delusions (often persecutory) and 'knight's move thinking'.
- Negative more chronic symptoms, such as lack of initiative and drive, poverty of speech, social withdrawal and isolation, poor self-care, blunt or flat affect, and impairment of cognitive function.

IV   Functional enquiry (FE)

The major purpose of the functional enquiry (or systems review) is to unearth symptoms of which the patient has not complained spontaneously and which he* (and perhaps you, until you are more knowledgeable) may feel are not relevant to the presenting complaint. Since the absence of certain symptoms as well as their presence is often helpful in diagnosis, these questions are asked in every case and the answer recorded whether positive or negative. In addition, this review forms part of the '1000 mile service'. Many of the questions may already have been asked and recorded during the HPC, and clearly they should not be repeated. If significant symptoms are identified during the functional enquiry, then further details are sought and recorded either under the appropriate section of the functional enquiry or another section of the history (for example, HPC, PMH, etc.).

Most experienced clinicians do not use such a check-list of symptoms to establish a diagnosis and formulate a plan of management. They tend to direct their questions specifically to the confirmation or rejection of a working diagnosis formulated during the initial history taking. In other words they tend to 'hunt' for the diagnosis by asking a limited number of questions relevant to the working diagnosis rather than acquiring a large amount of information from which to base a diagnosis and plan management ('trawling').

However, it is important that the functional enquiry is used to the full in the early stages of clinical medicine because:

- Asking about all the important symptoms gives you a 'feel' for them and serves as a reminder of them.
- You may not recognise the full importance of a symptom in diagnosis and assessment.
- A recorded negative response to a particular question may be useful if the patient presents in the future.

In the scheme that follows, the questions that are asked routinely are given under their appropriate system headings. If the response is positive then additional questions that should be asked to define the positive answer are given. There is then a brief outline of the significance of these symptoms with some of the more important being discussed in more detail. It is clear that only when you have more detailed knowledge of the medical conditions involved can you be very detailed in your questioning, but it is also clear that this section cannot be comprehensive in its discussion of the significance of symptoms. Reference to a standard medical text is important.

1   General

- *Fatigue*

- *Malaise*
  Pyrexia, rigors, night sweats

- *Sleep disturbance*
  Difficulty in getting to sleep
  Early waking
  Snoring
  Reduction in total number of hours asleep
  Reduced quality of sleep (not refreshing)

- *Skin*
  Rashes – distribution, itching, blistering, pain, bleeding
  Bruising
  Colour

- *Hair*
  Too much or too little
  Coarse or fine
  Abnormal distribution (particularly women)

Fatigue

This is a very common and non-specific symptom. Most patients will say at some stage in the interview 'Oh, and I always feel so tired'. Document what he* is unable to do because of lethargy with regard to work, leisure, hobbies, housework. Enquire about features of depression (a common cause of fatigue) and then consider diagnoses such as anaemia, hypothyroidism, or heart failure. Patients will sometimes ascribe the onset of fatigue to a viral illness – Post Viral Fatigue Syndrome or Myalgic Encephalomyelitis (ME).

Malaise

This is a feeling of being unwell with no specific features although symptoms such as fever or loss of appetite may accompany the feeling. Malaise is a feature of many physical and psychiatric illnesses and may even be the presenting complaint. Further detailed questioning is important to try to establish the system (or systems) involved so that physical examination and investigation may be pointed in this direction.

Night sweats, fevers, rigors

Because of the diurnal variation of temperature (maximum at about 10 p.m. and minimum at 2 a.m.) it is not uncommon for sweating to occur (to increase heat loss) in the early hours of the morning (night sweat) as a normal phenomenon. Change in body temperature will be felt as alternating between being cold and shivery (as temperature increases), hot with headache (at maximum temperature) and sweating (as heat is lost and temperature falls).

Rigor is the term applied to rapid increase in temperature associated with violent shivering and a feeling of intense cold. Malaria is the classical cause of rigor but it may be caused by sudden release of pyrogens from any source such as infected gall bladder or pyelonephritis.

It is important to document whether the above symptoms are indeed associated with significantly elevated body temperature because fever is a symptom (not a diagnosis) the underlying cause of which should be found.

Pyrexia (or fever) of unknown origin (PUO or FUO) refers to an illness characterised by prolonged fever (usually longer than 10 days so as to exclude self-limiting conditions such as viral infections) the cause of which is uncertain despite basic investigation (which will include urine culture and chest radiograph). The formal definition is an illness with fever exceeding 38.3°C, evolving during at least 3 weeks, with no diagnosis reached after 1 week of investigation.

Diagnosis depends on detailed history and repeated full clinical examination in addition to more specialised investigations.

Causes include:

- Infections (such as tuberculosis).
- Malignancy (such as lymphoma and renal carcinoma).
- Diseases with an immunological basis such as collagen vascular diseases (for example systemic lupus erythematosis).
- Others such as drug reaction (drug fever), inflammatory bowel

disease and factitious fever where a patient uses subterfuge to simulate an illness with fever.

Computed tomography of the abdomen is a very valuable investigation as it clearly demonstrates retroperitoneal structures such as enlarged lymph nodes.

In up to 25% of patients no diagnosis is made despite extensive investigation.

Sleep disturbance

Difficulty in getting to sleep may be due to anxiety and early morning waking is a feature of depression. Excessive snoring which is usually mentioned by the partner (or sometimes next-door neighbour!) rather than the patient is a feature of obstructive sleep apnoea syndrome particularly if there are short periods where breathing stops altogether to be followed by snorting and arousal so that sleep is very restless. The patient may wake with a headache due to carbon dioxide retention and will tend to be very drowsy during the day, falling asleep very readily. It is important to be alert to this diagnosis because chronic nocturnal hypoxia leads to pulmonary hypertension and cor pulmonale; acute hypoxia may cause fatal arrhythmias; and also, because such people are at risk from road traffic accidents (and other trauma) if they fall asleep in inappropriate situations, such as while driving.

Establish that poor quality of sleep is not due to a medical cause the symptoms of which always seem worse at night – for example breathlessness due to pulmonary or cardiac disease; palpitation; pain and discomfort related to cancer or arthritis; or nocturia from any cause. Patients with hyperthyroidism will tend to be hyperactive and sleep less. The commonest acute medical disorder which interferes with sleep is upper respiratory tract viral infection leading to sore throat and blocked nose.

The elderly seem to require less sleep at night (but may 'cat-nap') during the day.

Caffeine and other stimulants will heighten arousal and prevent sleep. Alcohol initially promotes sleep (which will be of poor quality) but will cause arousal (often with tachycardia) in the early hours of the morning due to release of catecholamines in the 'withdrawal' phase.

Skin

It is important to establish where a skin rash first appeared and its current distribution. For example:

Photosensitive eruptions tend to occur on light-exposed areas such as face, the 'V' of the neck and forearms;

Acne vulgaris has a distribution that involves the face, shoulders and back;

Contact dermatitis affects areas (particularly hands) exposed to the causative agent;

Psoriasis tends to affect the extensor surfaces of the limbs (particularly elbows and knees).

Itching (pruritus) is an important feature of many skin disorders. Scabies, insect bites, eczema and dermatitis herpetiformis are intensely itchy while psoriasis (for example) tends not to be. Itching is also a feature of non-dermatological conditions (where there is no primary skin rash) such as obstructive jaundice, renal failure or lymphoma. It is important to remember that many drugs will cause pruritus with or without a skin rash.

Skin colour may be altered by hypo- or hyper-pigmentation and this may be localised or generalised. Generalised hyper-pigmentation occurs as a racial feature and after ultra-violet light exposure (tanning) in addition to conditions such as Addison's disease (adrenal failure), renal failure and haemochromatosis. Localised hyper-pigmentation is seen in neurofibromatosis (*café-au-lait* patches), acanthosis nigricans (particularly of the axilla) and secondary to chronic inflammation of any cause.

Generalised hypo-pigmentation is a feature of albinism and is also seen in hypopituitarism. Localised hypo-pigmentation occurs in vitiligo (an immune destruction of the melanocytes associated with other auto-immune conditions such as diabetes mellitus, Addison's disease and pernicious anaemia), leprosy, localised scleroderma and is associated with scarring from any cause.

Blistering skin rashes include eczema, pemphigus and pemphigoid.

Hair

Change in quantity, quality or distribution of hair suggests an endocrine disorder. In hypothyroidism the hair will become sparse and coarse, and women who develop androgen producing tumours will develop male-pattern hair distribution. Excessive hair growth is often racial and familial and seen particularly in women from the Indian subcontinent.

2   Cardiovascular system (CVS)

- *Chest pain*
  Standard questions for pain (see HPC and below)

- *Shortness of breath (SOB)*
  True breathlessness
  Assessment of severity (exercise tolerance)
  Duration
  Wheeze
  Constant (predictable with exertion) or intermittent
  Relation to seasons, work, time of day or night, position
  Precipitating factors such as exercise, coughing, excitement,
      pain, lying flat (how many pillows?)
  Procedures and treatment which relieve breathlessness

- *Palpitation*
  Frequency, duration of attacks
  Whether they start and stop suddenly
  Pulse rate and rhythm during an attack (ask patient to tap out
      the rate and rhythm)
  Occasional 'missed beats'
  Provoking or relieving factors
  Associated symptoms such as breathlessness, chest pain or
      faintness

- *Swelling of legs*
  Duration
  Whether present after a night's rest
  Presence of varicose veins
  One leg or both legs affected
  Legs painful

Chest pain

It is useful to use the check-list for PAIN (see HPC, p. 11) to describe cardiac ischaemia.

Site	Central chest, anywhere between mandible and xiphisternum – occasionally upper abdomen.
Radiation	Either or both arms to finger tips (often inside of left arm), jaw.
Severity	Very severe, often associated with vomiting and sweating and requiring opiates for relief. A feeling of anxiety makes the discomfort worse.
Character	Not usually described as 'pain' but rather 'discomfort', constricting, strangling and often demonstrated with a clenched fist.

Onset	Gradually increasing over minutes.
Duration	A few minutes to several hours depending upon whether infarction or angina.
Frequency	Angina may occur many times a day depending upon circumstances.
Periodicity	Angina lacks periodicity although tends to improve in summer and with medication and reversal of risk factors.
Precipitating factors	Anything which will increase the work load of the heart (in angina) – exercise (particularly after a meal), emotion, meals, extremes of temperature particularly cold wind.
Relieving factors	Anything which reduces the work load of the heart (in angina) – rest, sublingual trinitrin.
Associated symptoms	Vomiting, breathlessness, malaise.

Cardiac pain lasting less than about 15 min and usually precipitated by exertion and other factors (reversible myocardial ischaemia) is called angina but more prolonged pain unassociated with precipitating cause should be considered as myocardial infarction (heart attack).

The pain of **pericarditis** is similar to cardiac ischaemic pain but tends to be relieved by sitting forward and may be intensified by swallowing or breathing.

Sudden onset of 'tearing' pain often precipitated by heavy lifting suggests **aortic pain**. The pain is very severe with radiation to the back between the shoulder blades. It may be associated with neurological symptoms and features of arterial occlusion if due to thoracic aortic dissection.

Chest pain may be due to **gastro-oesophageal disease** since the heart and the oesophagus have common innervation. In addition, it is clear that there is a viscerocardiac reflex which leads to constriction of the coronary arteries when the lower oesophagus is stimulated ('linked angina').

Shortness of breath (SOB)

Dyspnoea is the subjective awareness of uncomfortable breathing. At rest the normal individual is unaware of his* breathing and any increase in ventilation which is appropriate for the metabolic demand of exercise is recognised as being due to the exertion, is not thought to be abnormal, and is not reported as breathlessness. The cause of dyspnoea is complex and involves central and peripheral mechanisms and often correlates poorly with the objective features (signs) of shortness of breath. Dyspnoea and fatigue are the two cardinal symptoms of cardiac failure but dyspnoea may also be due to respiratory disease or to conditions such as anaemia.

Establish that breathlessness is not:

- 'Cannot get enough air', a feeling of smothering, or the need to get fresh air – symptoms which suggest anxiety and panic attacks.
- Chest tightness which may be angina
- Due to chest wall or pleuritic pain

Quantify the breathlessness by describing what the patient is able to do as follows:

- SOB at rest
- SOB on minimal exertion such as dressing
- Able to walk at own pace on flat ground
- Able to walk with spouse/dog on flat ground
- Able to walk up an incline/flight of stairs (state number of stairs)
- Able to carry shopping/lift light items

Remember that unfit individuals and those with sedentary jobs will have a limited exercise tolerance, and those with arthritis or angina may be limited by these problems rather than by dyspnoea.

Establish whether the dyspnoea is:

- Predictable with exertion (chronic obstructive pulmonary disease)
- Variable with time, treatment or precipitating factors (asthma, anxiety).

Orthopnoea is breathlessness which occurs on lying flat and is usually a feature of heart failure but may be due to obesity or bilateral diaphragmatic paralysis.

Quantitate by asking whether the patient has to be propped up (on how many pillows) to go to sleep, or whether he* has to sleep in a chair. Ensure that it is breathlessness itself (rather than pain or discomfort due to arthritis for example) that requires him* to be propped up and ask what happens if he* slides down the bed during the night. Some patients say that they are more comfortable sleeping propped up but as they do not become breathless when they slip down they do not have orthopnoea.

When the patient has **paroxysmal nocturnal dyspnoea (PND)** he* awakes suddenly in the early hours of the morning gasping for breath and may produce pink, frothy sputum due to pulmonary oedema. He* sits up with legs hanging over the side of the bed or stands by the window taking deep breaths of air. Symptoms subside within 30 min or so or are more prolonged and require emergency treatment.

When the patient is upright during the day there is about 500 ml blood pooled in the legs. This volume is returned to the circulation on lying down and causes cardiac decompensation if there is poor myocardial reserve. In addition, when the patient is lying down the hydrostatic pressure in the left atrium is increased and this contributes to the production of acute pulmonary oedema (left ventricular failure).

Bronchial asthma is also a cause of nocturnal breathlessness and cough and should not be confused with PND (also called 'cardiac asthma').

Palpitation

Normally the beating of the heart is not appreciated and palpitation is an unpleasant awareness of the heart's action. This may be due to a change in rhythm, rate or force of contraction, or a combination of these.

Swelling of legs

Swelling of one leg suggests local venous or lymphatic insufficiency or infection of the skin (cellulitis). The presence of pain is important and suggests deep venous thrombosis, cellulitis, rupture of a popliteal (Baker's) cyst or muscle trauma.

Swelling of both legs may be due to heart failure where an increase in right atrial pressure is transmitted to the peripheral veins; thrombosis of the inferior vena cava (when there will be little diurnal change in the amount of swelling), or low plasma oncotic pressure due to low serum albumin (nephrotic syndrome or cirrhosis of the liver).

3   Respiratory system (RS)

- *Shortness of breath*
  As in CVS (see p. 33)
  Association with wheezing, cough, sputum

- *Chest pain*
  Increased by breathing (pleuritic)
  Constant

- *Cough*
  Duration

First thing in the morning (matutinal), or all day
Painful and associated with other upper respiratory tract
    symptoms
Precipitating factors such as cold, exercise, posture
Associated phenomena such as wheezing, pain, regurgitation
Procedures which relieve cough

- Sputum
Amount (e.g. eggcupful)
Colour
Viscidity
Postural drainage

- Haemoptysis
Duration
Whether frank blood or mixed with sputum
Relationship to severe coughing bout
Associated with chest pain

Asthma is defined as a chronic inflammatory disorder of the airways that causes widespread but variable airflow obstruction that is often reversible spontaneously, or with treatment, and causes an associated increase in airway responsiveness to a variety of stimuli. It is a common condition and causes wheezing, breathlessness, chest tightness and cough with sputum production. These symptoms occur in susceptible individuals in attacks provoked by allergens (pollen, animal dander), inhaled irritants, exercise or viral infections. Nocturnal breathlessness and cough are particularly characteristic and should not be confused with PND.

Cough

Cough is a very important reflex which protects the airway from inhalation of pharyngeal or gastric secretions and foreign bodies which may cause aspiration pneumonia or bronchial obstruction and lung collapse.

Receptors in the large airways and larynx are stimulated by:

- Inflammatory mediators
- Mechanical injury
- Thermal and chemical irritation

These triggers activate the effector side of the reflex. Often the receptors are sensitised by one of the above mechanisms (such as viral infection) and so respond more readily to another (inhalation of cold air, dust particles, etc.). Angiotensin-converting enzyme inhibitors (ACEI) used in the treatment of heart failure and hypertension sensitise the airway (possibly by preventing the destruction of kinins) and cause a very irritating dry cough. Stimulation of the efferent limb causes the glottis to close, the intrathoracic pressure to increase and when the glottis is then relaxed air is forcibly expelled.

- No cough is normal – the 'normal' smokers' cough is the earliest feature of chronic bronchitis.
- Acute cough (a few days) is typical of viral infection.
- Chronic cough may be due to chronic bronchitis (defined as a cough productive of sputum occurring each day for 3 months for 2 consecutive years), bronchiectasis or lung cancer.
- Morning (matutinal) cough suggests chronic bronchitis or post-nasal drip; nocturnal cough suggests asthma or aspiration of gastric or pharyngeal contents.
  The description of the cough may be important in determining its cause:
  - barking cough is laryngeal in origin;
  - brassy is tracheal or originating in a major airway;
  - bovine implies vocal cord paralysis often from recurrent laryngeal nerve palsy;
  - a weak cough is seen in bilateral vocal cord palsy, respiratory muscle weakness and severe debility from any cause.

Associated features include syncope, rib fracture and pneumothorax.

Sputum

The mucus glands which line the bronchial tree produce approximately 100 ml clear mucus in 24 hours. The mucus is driven towards the larynx by the action of the bronchial cilia (muco-ciliary 'escalator') and is usually swallowed. Irritation of the bronchial tree causes an increase in the production of mucus and this is coughed up (expectorated) as clear white tenacious (mucoid) sputum.

When there is bacterial infection of the bronchial tree the mucus contains pus cells which cause the sputum to become thinner and yellow. Verdoperoxidase changes the colour to green and this green/yellow sputum is termed 'purulent'. Eosinophils in the sputum (which may be present in asthma) give the same appearance but the sputum is tenacious.

Mucous plugs or casts of the bronchial tree may be seen in the sputum of patients with asthma.

The daily production of sputum should be quantitated (eggcup, teacup, etc.) and enquiries made as to the position in which most sputum is expectorated (postural drainage). Large volumes of sputum suggest bronchiectasis and the position of the patient that encourages the greatest production of sputum helps to locate the area of lung which is affected.

Haemoptysis is the term given to expectorated blood.

It may be:

- A fresh streak in mucoid sputum which suggests lung cancer;
- Rusty in colour due to alveolar blood from pneumonia;
- Frank blood which may be due to tuberculosis or pulmonary infarction
- Or false due to vomiting of blood (the liquid is bitter) or blood from the nasopharynx (which tastes salty).

Despite investigation (including bronchoscopy) no cause is found to explain about half the cases of haemoptysis.

Chest pain

May originate from:

- *The pleura*
  The lung parenchyma and visceral pleura have no pain receptors and lesions within the lung are painless. When there is extension of inflammation, or infection to the periphery of the lung, the parietal pleura is involved and pleuritic pain (pleurisy) occurs. This pain is typically increased on inspiration and limits the depth of respiration as if the two inflamed surfaces are rubbing against each other and causing pain. Pneumonia, pulmonary infarction (following pulmonary embolus) and inflammatory conditions of the pleura (collagen diseases) may cause pleuritic pain.

- *The diaphragm*
  This pain is usually pleuritic in nature and referred to the shoulder.

- *The chest wall (ribs, spine, intercostal muscles)*
  This is a constant pain which tends to increase on inspiration and also with movement and position.

- *The costo-chondral junctions*
  Presumed inflammation of the costal cartilages (costochondritis) causes constant chest pain and local tenderness. This tends to be

described as Tietze syndrome but this term is best reserved for a condition in which the costo-chondral junction is truly inflamed (swollen and warm), rather than just tender.

4   Alimentary system (AS)

- *Appetite*
  Normal, or reduced
  If reduced, is it due to anorexia or pain/discomfort associated with eating or dysphagia
  Associated weight loss

- *Difficulty in swallowing (dysphagia)*
  Due to pain in mouth (e.g. aphthous ulcers) or difficulty with mastication
  Progressive or intermittent
  Solids or liquids more affected
  Site where food lodges/sticks

- *Heartburn*
  Precipitating factors such as tight corsets, bending forwards, lying down

- *Abdominal pain*
  Standard questions for pain (see HPC, p. 11)

- *Bowels*
  Regular or irregular
  Change in habit
  Diarrhoea
  Constipation
  Urgency, incontinence, tenesmus
  Steatorrhoea
  Melaena

- *Nausea*

- *Vomiting*
  Regurgitation or true vomiting
  Effortless, projectile, self-induced
  Quantity, colour, constituents

Blood
Frequency, time of day or night
Relation to meals, coughing, drug ingestion

● *Indigestion, dyspepsia*
  Determine exactly what is meant e.g. loss of appetite,
    flatulence, heartburn, regurgitation, feeling of fullness,
    nausea, vomiting, abdominal pain, etc.

Anorexia

This is a lack of desire to eat, or loss of appetite. Make sure that it is not the fear of eating because of pain, which limits food intake.

Anorexia is a non-specific symptom but may suggest gastric (e.g. carcinoma), or hepatic (e.g. secondary malignancy or hepatitis) abnormality.

Anorexia nervosa is a condition in which there appears to be a morbid fear of weight gain and patients (usually girls) will starve themselves, or repeatedly gorge and vomit (bulimia), to limit their calorie intake.

Diagnostic criteria for anorexia nervosa include:

● Refusal to maintain body weight at, or above, a minimum normal weight calculated for age and height.
● Intense fear of gaining weight, or becoming fat, despite being underweight.
● Disturbance of body image in that being underweight is still appreciated as being too fat and the seriousness of current low body weight is denied.
● Three consecutive months of amenorrhoea.

Dysphagia

This is difficulty in swallowing, or an awareness that there is something wrong with the mechanism of swallowing, a symptom which must always be taken seriously. There may be pain or discomfort that is difficult to localise. Any painful lesion of the mouth such as aphthous ulcer or dental abscess may cause dysphagia.

Aphthous ulcers involve the buccal mucosa or tongue. They start as small white/grey, very painful nodules which may ulcerate interfering with eating and drinking, but heal within a few days. They are commoner in women, in relation to menstruation, and they may appear after dental treatment. In some patients, they may be associated with malabsorption syndrome such as coeliac disease or Crohn's disease and ulcerative colitis.

In other patients difficulty, or pain, is experienced when swallowing begins and the food bolus passes through the pharynx which is inflamed due to tonsillitis for example. The mouth may be too dry to enable swallowing, or there may be a neurological disorder of the pharynx or muscles of mastication.

Dysphagia may be:

- Mechanical, such as in carcinoma of the oesophagus. There is relentless progression with difficulty first noted for solid food and then liquids.
- Neurological, when there is abnormality of the normal oesophageal motility. Dysphagia is often noted first for liquids and there may be regurgitation and aspiration into the lung causing cough and lung abscess.

Finally, some patients may have difficulty in swallowing because of anxiety ('lump in the throat'), which is referred to as **globus hystericus** and is not associated with demonstrable abnormality.

Heartburn

Burning epigastric pain that radiates retrosternally and up to the throat is due to reflux of gastric acid into the oesophagus. It may be associated with hiatus hernia (this may be demonstrated by barium meal or by endoscopy), or with incompetence of the cardiac sphincter of the stomach without obvious hernia. Acid reflux may cause inflammation of the lower oesophagus (oesophagitis) and lead to stricture formation – gastro-oesophageal reflux disease (GORD).

Abdominal pain

May be:

- Visceral due to stretching of a viscus or tension on the mesentery. It is dull and poorly localised, usually to the midline. Visceral pain may originate from:

    Oesophagus – substernal
    Stomach or duodenum – epigastric
    Small intestine – periumbilical
    Colon – lower mid abdominal
    Gall bladder – epigastrium and right upper quadrant
    Pancreas – epigastrium radiating through to back

- Parietal when the parietal peritoneum is involved in an inflammatory process. The pain is intense, localised and made worse by movement and coughing.
- Referred

Nausea

This is defined as an unpleasant sensation, which suggests that vomiting is imminent but may not occur even after long periods of nausea. There is associated anorexia and also physiological changes, which include salivation, increased swallowing, sweating, pallor and tachycardia. The mechanism whereby the actual sensation of nausea is produced is unknown and the causes of nausea are those which also cause vomiting.

Vomiting

The vomiting centre in the brainstem receives impulses from:

- The upper gastrointestinal tract mainly via the vagus nerve. Mechanoreceptors respond to distension (in intestinal obstruction for example) and chemoreceptors are activated by chemical irritants such as bacterial toxins and alcohol in the gut lumen.
- The chemoreceptor trigger zone in the floor of the fourth ventricle which is outside the 'blood-brain barrier' and can respond to circulating emetic substances such as morphine. This centre may also respond to increased intracranial pressure to produce vomiting.
- The vestibular system (semicircular canals and otolith organs) which is responsible for the symptoms of motion sickness. In addition, this system may be involved in pathological processes such as viral infection (vestibular neuronitis) and Menière's disease, which will cause the same symptoms.
- Cerebral pathways which cause nausea and vomiting in response to a repulsive sight or smell.

Haematemesis is the vomiting of blood, the source of which will be the stomach or duodenum (usually above the ligament of Trietz). This must be distinguished from blood which is swallowed (from the nose or pharynx) and subsequently vomited.

Frank blood is recognised in the vomitus as dark red clots. If the blood is partially digested by acid it appears as 'coffee grounds'. So that the diagnosis of haematemesis is not inappropriately made too frequently, it is important to realise that watery stomach contents frequently contain dark particles that are not flecks of blood, and that stick-testing for blood is often positive in the absence of clinically significant haemorrhage.

Upper gastrointestinal bleeding is a common clinical problem. In over 80% of patients the bleeding will settle spontaneously but the other patients require intensive support and surgery, and the patients in this group have a significant mortality which has changed little over the last 30 years despite advances in management.

The haemodynamic effects of haemorrhage will depend on the amount of blood lost, and will tend to be more severe in the elderly and in those with medical conditions such as ischaemic heart disease, heart failure and chronic lung disease. A major bleed is one where the patient is hypotensive with a tachycardia and is pale and shocked. Such patients will have lost up to 40% of their circulating blood volume. Less severe blood loss (15–20% of blood volume) will cause persistent tachycardia and postural hypotension. Minor bleeding will not have any effect on the circulation but may anticipate future major blood loss, particularly when the cause of the bleeding is oesophageal varices.

Causes of haematemesis include:

- Oesophageal mucosal tear particularly after violent vomiting (Mallory-Weiss).
- Duodenal ulcer or gastric ulcer eroding into an artery.
- Erosive gastritis or duodenitis often caused by drugs such as aspirin and other non-steroidal anti-inflammatory drugs or alcohol.
- Oesophageal varices caused by cirrhosis of the liver and portal hypertension.
- Carcinoma of the stomach.

Bile-stained (green) vomit implies that there is no pyloric obstruction. Large volumes of vomit often containing recognisable food from previous meals characteristically occur in gastric outflow obstruction due to either stricture from chronic peptic ulceration or gastric carcinoma.

Bowels

Melaena refers to the black, tarry appearance of blood altered by digestion in the stools which have a typically pungent smell. The origin of the blood is usually the stomach and duodenum often in association with haematemesis. Occasionally, the blood may arise from a more distal site in the bowel but if there is no opportunity for digestion to occur it appears in the rectum as frank blood. Bleeding from the stomach or duodenum may be so brisk that the rapid transit through the bowel does not allow for significant digestion of the blood to occur and the blood appears in the rectum largely unchanged, rather than as melaena.

Steatorrhoea is diarrhoea due to fat malabsorption. The stools are beige or putty coloured and typically float in the lavatory pan and are difficult to flush away (this is due to the trapped gas rather than to the increased fat content itself). Conditions causing fat malabsorption include coeliac disease (where there will also tend to be malabsorption of folic acid and iron) and obstructive jaundice (due to gallstones, carcinoma of the pancreas or primary biliary cirrhosis), which is accompanied by dark bile-stained urine.

Diarrhoea is defined as a daily stool weight of 200 gm or more, and is usually associated with stools that are more fluid and passed more frequently than usual.

Abnormality of the small intestine causes large volume stools, which are watery, foul-smelling and may contain undigested food. There may be periumbilical discomfort.

Abnormality of the colon causes small stools with urgency of defaecation and tenesmus (the uncomfortable feeling that the rectum has not been completely emptied). The stool may contain blood or mucus (slime) and be associated with lower abdominal pain.

Constipation refers to stools that are too hard, too small, too difficult to expel (straining) or passed too infrequently. This traditional definition is difficult to interpret because the normal range is not known and each patient may have a different attitude towards his* bowel function (some older people are brought up to expect daily defecation as a measure of 'inner cleanliness'). Fewer than three defecations a week is generally accepted as being abnormal, but some people defecate only once or twice a week and have no symptoms. Vegetarians pass bulkier stools than meat eaters, and a change in diet may lead to a change in bowel habit (for example, regular beer drinkers may become constipated when they do not drink for a few days). Some people will not defecate because they do not have time in the mornings, have a lack of toilet facilities or suppress a call to stool for social reasons.

It may be better to define constipation according to the appearance and form of the stool with separate round lumps (like nuts) being a definitely constipated stool and a sausage-shaped but lumpy stool being suggestive of constipation. It is the change of bowel habit which is important.

Flatulence

Establish whether this is a feeling of fullness and bloating ('wind'), or the passage of gas 'northwards or southwards'.

Belching is due to air swallowing and is of social rather than medical importance.

Flatus is the passage of gas per rectum. The gas is derived from the fermentation of carbohydrate in the bowel and excess flatus (difficult to define) may suggest malabsorption or bacterial overgrowth. Most commonly, it is associated with a diet which is high in fibre.

Dyspepsia

This non-specific term includes episodic or persistent symptoms that are likely to arise in the proximal gastrointestinal tract such as epigastric pain and discomfort, post prandial fullness, bloating, belching, nausea, anorexia, heart burn and regurgitation. These symptoms may be grouped into three main categories, which suggest a cause as follows:

- *Gastro-oesophageal reflux disease (GORD)*
  Heartburn and regurgitation

- *Peptic ulcer (PU)*
  Localised epigastric pain
  Nocturnal pain
  Relief obtained from antacids, food, vomiting

- *Irritable bowel syndrome (IBS)/dysmotility*
  Poorly localised discomfort
  Fullness after small meals
  Bloating
  Nausea

Patients over the age of 45 yr who present with the above symptoms may require further investigation (such as upper gastrointestinal endoscopy) to exclude other causes of dyspepsia, particularly if they also have dysphagia, persistent vomiting, weight loss, bleeding or anaemia.

Irritable bowel syndrome (IBS) is a symptom complex in which the most frequent symptoms are abdominal pain and bloating. In addition, there is frequently alternating constipation and diarrhoea, the latter typically occurring after meals (particularly breakfast) and sometimes associated with urgency. Motility studies of the bowel show that there is abnormal contractility that corresponds to pain, and that when a balloon is distended in the gut of a patient with IBS the distension required to produce pain is less than normal. The symptoms however, correlate poorly with these objective measures and patients who come to medical attention tend to have an abnormal psychological state which may increase their awareness of these symptoms.

5   Genito-urinary system (GUS)

- *Micturition*
  Burning pain on passing water (dysuria)
  Number of times bladder emptied during the day (frequency)
  Passing large volumes of urine (polyuria)
  Drinking abnormally large volumes of fluids (polydipsia)
  Urgent desire to empty bladder (urgency)
  Oliguria
  Incontinence

- *Symptoms of prostatism (in men)*
  Difficulty in starting micturition
  Poor stream (are you able to hit the wall or back of the pan?)
  Dribbling at the end of micturition (terminal dribbling)
  Number of times bladder emptied at night (nocturia)

- *Urine colour*
  Dark (like tea)
  *Red due to presence of blood (haematuria), haemoglobin
    (haemoglobinuria), coloured pigment (e.g. beetroot)*

- *Renal pain*

Micturition

Dysuria refers to burning or painful sensation before, during, or after micturition although in its widest sense it may refer to any difficulty with bladder voiding. It may be associated with blood in the urine and increased frequency of micturition, with the passing of small volumes of urine and urgency (symptoms of cystitis). The usual cause is bladder infection, but urethral inflammation without infection is also common, particularly in women.

Frequency is defined as the number of times the bladder is emptied during the day. However, it is usually taken to mean abnormally increased frequency with the passage of small volumes of urine, often associated with symptoms of cystitis.

Polyuria is an increase in the total daily volume of urine. This is usually manifest by an increased frequency of micturition (including the night – nocturia) but with the passing of large volumes of urine. Voiding during the day more frequently than every 2 hours and voiding more than twice at night in those under the age of about 50 yr is abnormal (unless there is excessive fluid intake). The cause may be a failure of concentrating power of the renal tubules, as in chronic renal failure or diabetes insipidus, or it may be due to the osmotic diuresis which occurs in diabetes mellitus and hypercalcaemia.

Nocturia occurs as a result of polyuria, and also in the elderly. The normal diurnal renal concentrating mechanism of the kidney leads to a reduction of urine volume during the night, and this is the first function to be affected by chronic renal disease and also old age. Nocturia is often the first symptom of the former, and a frequent association of the latter.

Nocturia is also a feature of prostatism; reduced bladder capacity and bladder inflammation; and also a consequence of drinking too much fluid (often alcohol) shortly before retiring to bed.

Oliguria is defined as a urine volume of less than 400 ml in 24 h. If no urine is passed the term is anuria. Oliguria is rarely a prominent symptom and it is usually apparent only when the urine volume is carefully measured. Oliguria suggests renal failure but may occur in severe dehydration, which may progress to renal failure if not corrected and must be distinguished from lower urinary tract obstruction (by ultrasound examination if necessary).

Urinary incontinence is the repeated involuntary loss of urine that constitutes a social or hygiene problem. It is a distressing symptom and one which may affect up to 5% of the general population and nearly 20% of those over the age of 65 yr. A useful classification is as follows:

- Stress incontinence
  Defined as the involuntary loss of urine due to an increase in intra-abdominal pressure in the absense of detrusor activity. It usually occurs in women, and is due to a deficiency in the urethral closure mechanism often associated with multiparity. Leakage of urine occurs with coughing, laughing, straining and physical exertion.
- Detrusor instability
  A condition in which the bladder detrusor muscle contracts during bladder filling even while the subject is attempting to inhibit micturition. In the majority of patients (usually women) no cause is found, but neurological disorders such as multiple sclerosis (MS) or spinal cord disruption may be implicated.

Bladder infection causes irritation of the trigone and this stimulates detrusor activity leading to urinary frequency and urgency of micturition with possible incontinence.

● Overflow

Bladder filling occurs to the point where the functional capacity is exceeded and incontinence results. This is often a feature of prostatic hypertrophy and bladder neck outflow obstruction.

● Lack of awareness or immobility

Patients with dementia and stroke are frequently incontinent of urine because of cognitive impairment. Those who are immobile due to arthritis (for example) may not be able to reach a toilet facility in time and so appear to be incontinent of urine. The prescription of powerful diuretics may exacerbate any tendency to bladder leakage.

Urine colour

Dark brown	–	bile associated with obstructive jaundice.
Smoky red	–	red cells suggesting glomerulonephritis
Bright red	–	haematuria due to bleeding anywhere in the renal tract
	–	haemoglobinuria due to haemolysis
	–	myoglobinuria due to muscle breakdown
	–	beeturia from eating beetroot
	–	from dyes present in food, often sweets such as peardrops

Renal pain

Pain from structural disease of the kidney is felt in the loin below the twelfth rib posteriorly as a dull ache. Gentle percussion over this area with your fist will exacerbate the pain.

Ureteric colic (not renal colic) is a very intense pain due to obstruction of the ureter with a stone or blood clot. It is true colic caused by spasm of the smooth muscle of the ureter and comes in waves with each bout of pain rising to a crescendo (when the patient writhes around in agony) and then fading over a few minutes. The pain radiates in the distribution of the nerve supply of the ureter from the renal angle round to the flank and then to the groin, penis or labia majora. The pain stops as soon as the obstruction is relieved, often with the passage of a stone per urethram.

- *Menstruation*
  Age of onset (menarche)
  Duration of bleeding and regularity recorded as K = 12,5/28
    (12 yr = menarche, 5/28 = 5 days blood loss every 28
    days)
  Heavy blood loss (menorrhagia)
  Painful periods (dysmenorrhoea)
  Infrequent periods (oligomenorrhoea)
  No periods (amenorrhoea)
  Associated symptoms such as fluid retention, painful breasts
  Intermenstrual bleeding (IMB)

- *Pain or discomfort on intercourse (dyspareunia)*

- *Menopause*
  Age when periods stopped recorded as K = 12,5/28,52
    (where 52 is the age of menopause)
  Post-menopausal bleeding (PMB)
  Hormone replacement therapy (HRT)

Menstruation

Menorrhagia is the complaint of excessive menstrual bleeding and objectively it is defined as blood loss greater than 80 ml per menstrual period, the mean normal blood loss being about 35 ml (90% is lost within the first three days). Menstrual blood loss is not routinely measured and symptoms that suggest menorrhagia are the passage of clots, flooding and requirement of extra sanitary protection (pads and tampons). However, it is often very difficult to assess accurately from the history the amount of blood loss and in hospital practice it was found that less than half of the number of women whose complaint was menorrhagia had a measured blood loss of greater than 80 ml. The presence of hypochromic, microcytic anaemia suggests excessive blood loss.

Intrauterine contraceptive devices (IUCD) are associated with increased menstrual blood loss. Women taking oral contraceptive pills frequently have very little menstrual blood loss.

Dysmenorrhoea is pain which coincides with menstruation and may be either:

- Primary, or spasmodic – this usually occurs in women before their first pregnancy in the early years of reproductive life and is associated with ovular rather than anovular menstrual cycles. It is attributed to the release of prostaglandins which cause vasoconstriction of the spiral arterioles of the uterus and painful myometrial contractions.

- Secondary – this is seen later in reproductive life and may be caused by endometriosis.

Oligomenorrhoea may herald approaching menopause but may be associated with endocrine abnormality such as polycystic ovary syndrome.

Amenorrhoea may be:

- Primary, when menstruation has never occurred and is often due to serious endocrine or structural abnormality. Investigation would not normally be undertaken until the age of about 17 yr.
- Secondary, when the menarche occurred normally but was followed by cessation of menstruation. Endocrine abnormalities particularly hyperprolactinaemia should be excluded but frequently the cause is psychological or related to weight loss or excessive physical training. The commonest cause is pregnancy!

Premenstrual syndrome (PMS): fluid retention, breast tenderness and mood swings are physiological features of the hormonal changes that occur in the normal menstrual cycle. In some women these are exaggerated and disabling, but it is not clear whether PMS is an entity or an exaggeration of the normal state.

Dyspareunia

This may be superficial and caused by vaginal or perineal problems (vaginal dryness due to oestrogen deficiency is probably the commonest cause), or deep when pelvic abnormality such as endometriosis should be suspected.

Menopause

This is defined as a woman's last menstrual period, and thus the end of her reproductive life. In practical terms it is impossible to say which is the last period until about 12 months have elapsed without menstruation. The mean age of the menopause in Western countries is 51.5 yr. The menopause may cause distressing symptoms of both a physical and psychological nature, which are due to oestrogen deficiency and possibly gonadotrophin excess. These symptoms include:

- Hot flushes, night sweats
- Urinary frequency/urgency and vaginal dryness, loss of libido.
- Insomnia, lethargy, irritability, depressed mood, loss of confidence and failure to cope with work and life.

In addition, the menopause is associated with an increased risk of vascular disease (particularly myocardial infarction) and osteoporosis. Early menopause may be familial, or due to premature ovarian failure and predicts the more rapid development of osteoporosis and premature vascular disease. Many women have hormone replacement therapy (HRT), which may be in the form of tablets or transdermal patches, not only to ameliorate menopausal symptoms but also to reduce the risk of bone loss and vascular disease.

Post-menopausal bleeding raises the possibility of uterine or vaginal malignancy and requires investigation usually with dilatation and curettage (D and C).

6   Central nervous system (CNS)

- *Right or left-handed*

- *Headache*
  Standard questions for pain (see HPC, p. 11)

- *Fits, faints, loss of consciousness, (LOC)*
  Frequency
  How long unconscious
  Description from witness particularly with regard to features of
      convulsion, facial colour, sweating, mode of recovery
  Incontinence, tongue biting or injury
  Funny or exceptional tastes, smells, feelings (aura)
  Preceded by symptoms of impending faint
  Related to change in posture

- *Vision*
  Corrected with spectacles
  Acuity
  Loss of vision (transient, focal, generalised)
  Double vision

- *Hearing (deafness)*
  Duration
  One or both ears
  Associated symptoms such as tinnitus, dizziness, vertigo

- *Vertigo, dizziness*

- *Weakness of limbs*
  Duration
  Onset and progression
  Focal or general, unilateral or bilateral, proximal or distal
  Unsteadiness, difficulty in walking, falls

- *Numbness, tingling (paraesthesiae)*
  Onset, duration and progression
  Distribution
  Provoking position

- *Personality changes*
  Apathy
  Irritable, aggressive

- *Loss of memory or concentration*

- *Smell, taste*

Headache

This is a very common symptom which is usually of little clinical significance. However, headache may reduce the ability to work and to enjoy social life and may be due to serious underlying conditions such as brain tumour. It is important to try and distinguish headache from facial pain and to beware of the self-diagnosis of 'migraine', which tends to be used by patients as a socially more acceptable term than 'headache'.

Migraine is divided into two main types:

1. Migraine without aura (80–90% of cases). This is defined as headache lasting 4–72 h (treated or untreated) with a headache-free interval between the attacks. There should be a history of at least five attacks. Each headache should have at least two of the following characteristics:
   - unilateral location
   - pulsating quality
   - moderate or severe intensity
   - aggravation by routine physical activity,
   and should be associated with at least one of the following symptoms:
   - nausea and/or vomiting
   - photophobia or phonophobia.

2. Migraine with aura (10–20% of cases). This is defined as above, but in addition, the headache is preceded by symptoms of transient (less than 60 min) focal cerebral, cortical or brain-stem dysfunction. The commonest symptom is visual disturbance consisting of homonymous impairment, or loss of vision, or bright flashing lights often in a zigzag formation with distortion of vision.

Cluster headaches (migrainous neuralgia) are very severe unilateral head pains lasting between 15 min and 3 h which occur in bouts (clusters) of several weeks separated by remissions lasting from months to years. Patients are usually young men.

Very sudden onset of severe headache (as if hit on the back of the head) associated with vomiting and photophobia suggests that a diagnosis of **subarachnoid haemorrhage** should be excluded (with CT brain scan or lumbar puncture).

Headache which is present particularly in the morning on waking suggests **raised intracranial pressure** (e.g. from cerebral tumour) or carbon dioxide retention associated with sleep apnoea syndrome. A common cause of matutinal headache is alcohol excess.

Headache which increases over hours and is associated with fever, photophobia and systemic upset should be assumed to be **meningitis** until proven otherwise.

Tension headache tends to increase as the day progresses and is associated with stiff painful neck muscles and hunched tense shoulders. Its quality may be described as bursting or 'like a band around the head', and is often located over the vertex. Symptoms of anxiety and depression are likely to be present. Abnormalities of the neck (cervical spondylosis) may cause muscle contraction headaches.

Dull, constant headache in an older person who also complains of scalp tenderness (as when brushing hair) may be due to **cranial arteritis** (temporal arteritis). There may be constitutional symptoms including anorexia, weight loss and fever and also aching and stiffness (but not weakness) of the proximal limb muscles (polymyalgia rheumatica). It is important to establish the diagnosis quickly and start treatment with corticosteroids as the arteritis may affect the ocular vessels leading to blindness.

Head pains may arise from teeth and sinuses and may be confused with 'headache'. Hypertension is not a cause of headache unless the blood pressure is greatly raised and refractive errors are unlikely to be the cause of headache, although patients will frequently seek the advice of the optician.

A general classification of headache and facial pain is shown in Table 1.

Table 1. *Classification of headache and facial pain*

Classification	Examples
Primary headache	
Migraine	Without aura
	With aura
Tension	
Cluster	
Miscellaneous	Exertional headache
	Cephalgia
	Cold
	Coitus
Secondary headache	
Post traumatic	Acute, chronic
Vascular disorders	Subarachnoid haemorrhage
	Cranial arteritis
Non-vascular intracranial	Meningitis
	Post-lumbar puncture
Toxic and drugs	Nitrates, alcohol
Systemic infection	Viral illness, pneumonia
Metabolic	Altitude
	Carbon dioxide retention
Neck disorders	Cervical spondylitis
Inflammatory cranial	Acute glaucoma
	Sinusitis
Cranial nerve disorders	Trigeminal neuralgia
	Post-herpetic neuralgia
Not classifiable	

Fits, faints, loss of consciousness

An **epileptic seizure** is a transient and intermittent disturbance of behaviour, emotion, motor function or sensation, which results from cortical neuronal discharge. **Epilepsy** is the term used when there are repeated seizures. An epileptic seizure occurs when the cortical neuronal excitatory stimuli outweigh the inhibitory stimuli, either because the seizure threshold is lowered for genetic or metabolic reasons, or because there is a structural abnormality (infarct, tumour etc.), which acts as a focus to disrupt neuronal function. Seizures are usually stereotyped in individuals and diagnosis depends on a detailed description of events from the patient himself* and from witnesses.

The following classification is used:

● *Partial seizures*

These have focal onset with motor, somatosensory, special sensory, autonomic or psychic symptoms and may be simple (with no loss of consciousness), or complex (where consciousness is impaired). A partial seizure may evolve into a tonic-clonic convulsion

● *Generalised seizures*

There is generalised onset with loss of consciousness and may be absence attack ('*petit mal*'), myoclonic, clonic, tonic-clonic ('*grand mal*') or atonic.

● *Status epilepticus*

Repetitive seizures occurring without the patient regaining consciousness. This is a medical emergency because frequent seizures can cause hypoxic brain damage.

The description of a **generalised tonic-clonic seizure** is very characteristic and diagnostic. It may start with an aura the details of which the patient may forget but it is clear to a witness that the subject is vacant and 'strange'. In addition, the patient may make preparations for the impending fit by moving away from furniture etc.

The tonic phase starts with sudden and very forceful contraction of all muscle groups and the patient falls rigid to the ground. He* may bite his* tongue (if it is between his* teeth), be incontinent of urine (if the bladder is full), injure himself* in the fall and the muscle contraction may even break a bone. Respiration stops and cyanosis develops causing great concern in the onlookers.

The clonic phase heralds stertorous respiration and relief of the cyanosis. There is generalised convulsing followed by a period of apparently peaceful sleep from which the patient appears to wake but is confused, drowsy and may have a headache.

On complete recovery the patient may remember nothing of the attack (except perhaps the aura), which is why an account from a witness is of vital importance and helps to distinguish epilepsy from other causes of loss of consciousness.

Syncope refers to loss of consciousness caused by temporary impairment of the cerebral circulation. The metabolism of the brain is highly dependent on perfusion, and cessation of cerebral blood flow leads to syncope within about 10 s.

Vasovagal syncope (or common faint) is the most common form. Peripheral vasodilatation occurs in response to a precipitating event and blood pressure tends to fall. Cardiac output fails to compensate because of relative bradycardia and blood pressure falls further, thus reducing cerebral perfusion. Syncope may occur particularly if the subject is standing, as blood will pool in the dependent parts.

Vasovagal syncope may be precipitated by a stressful or painful experience and is more likely to occur in association with hunger, fatigue or being in a crowded place, particularly when standing in a hot room. The vasodilator effect of alcohol is additive (cocktail party). Premonitory signs and symptoms are common and are usually summed up by the patient as 'feeling awful'. These include pallor, sweating, nausea, hyperventilation, blurred vision and a vague feeling of unawareness as if everything was going on at a distance. If the patient sits (or preferably lies down) then frank syncope may be prevented but otherwise consciousness is lost. Cerebral perfusion returns when the patient assumes (involuntarily) the lying position, but recovery is often slow with continued nausea and 'unwellness'. It is not uncommon for patients to feel unwell for many hours after a severe episode.

Micturition syncope is the term given to syncope which occurs when the full bladder is emptied. It is usually a problem of elderly men who have nocturia due to prostatic enlargement. They get out of a warm bed in the early hours of the morning and stand at the lavatory. Blood pressure will tend to be low under these circumstances and may be further reduced by the Valsalva manoeuvre produced by straining. However, it is the autonomic discharge associated with bladder emptying which precipitates the fall in blood pressure that causes syncope.

Adams-Stokes attacks produce sudden loss of consciousness due to episodes of asystole usually associated with heart block. The patient becomes unconscious, 'deathly pale' and limp without warning. Complete and rapid recovery occurs after a few seconds, with colour returning as a flush as the circulation is restored. Urgent investigation is required with a view to pacemaker insertion.

Vision

The commonest cause of reduced visual acuity (poorly able to read or watch the television) which is not corrected by spectacles is **cataract**. **Glaucoma** may cause painless and insidious visual loss.

Left **hemianopia** (often as a result of stroke) may present as difficulty in reading as the start of each new line is not appreciated (when reading from left to right). In addition, patients may bump into the left side of doorframes and drive into parked cars (when driving on the left).

Amaurosis fugax is sudden and transient loss of vision in one eye. It is a very specific form of transient ischaemic attack (TIA) and implies atheromatous disease of the ipsilateral carotid artery.

Diplopia (or double vision) suggests an abnormality of the extra-ocular muscles or their cranial nerves and central connections and will prompt careful neurological examination.

Vertigo, dizziness

Vertigo is the feeling of rotation – the patient senses rotation of either himself* or his* surroundings. It may be accompanied by unsteadiness (reduced coordination) or deafness and tinnitus (suggesting a middle-ear problem such as Menière's disease).

Dizziness is a common symptom and one which needs to be defined by careful questioning. It may refer to true vertigo; a feeling of light-headedness (often due to hyperventilation and anxiety); unsteadiness from a variety of causes; headache; or 'muzziness' which is very non-specific.

7   Locomotor system

- *Ask about joints:*
  Pain, stiffness or swelling of the joints
  Distribution of affected joints
  Morning stiffness
  Pain relieved by rest and worse on weight-bearing
  Functional capacity

- *Ask about limb weakness*
  As in CNS (p. 53)

Arthralgia is the term used to describe pain and stiffness of joints, but where there is also swelling or other evidence of inflammation the term is **arthritis**. Pain and stiffness which is worse in the morning and takes several hours to 'loosen up' is characteristic of inflammatory conditions such as rheumatoid arthritis and ankylosing spondylitis. In mechanical disorders such as osteoarthritis the pain and stiffness are aggravated by exercise and are worst at the end of the day.

It is important to document the degree of disability that the joint problems cause and this may vary from almost full mobility to being confined to a wheelchair. Ask about ability to do gardening, household duties and shopping as well as problems with dressing and personal hygiene. Ask also what assistance is available and what aids are used.

8 Minimal statement of functional enquiry

This should include a positive or negative statement about every question listed under each system (see checklist on p. 176.)

9 Initial differential diagnosis

Although not traditionally taught it is very helpful to compose a list of possible diagnoses at the end of the interview and before continuing with the physical examination. This initial differential diagnosis will help you decide what are important positive and negative points to be discovered on further enquiry or examination. It will allow you to concentrate on confirming or excluding any of these diagnoses and enable you to give emphasis to certain parts of your structured clinical examination.

V Physical examination

1 Introduction

At all stages of the physical examination you must ensure the patient's privacy and comfort. Explain to him* what you are going to do in simple terms which are easily understood both at the beginning and again at appropriate stages of examination. It is better to say for example 'turn towards me' rather than 'turn onto your right side'. Remember particularly that what may be routine for you, may be new, embarrassing, or uncomfortable for the patient.

You are about to observe and lay hands upon a stranger who will have on few clothes, may be feeling unwell, and who will therefore be very vulnerable and insecure. It is important that you have a kind, courteous and professional attitude and also have clean, warm hands and tidy hair. Many elderly patients will object to designer stubble and earrings (on men!) or drooping hair, and this objection should be respected. The room should be warm and only the area to be examined should be exposed at any one time. The patient should be asked to change position as little as possible (sitting up, lying down or turning to one side) during the examination. Disposable gloves are appropriate for the examination of areas such as the mouth or genitalia, and weeping or infected skin lesions.

It is usual to look initially at the patient in general terms and collect together signs such as anaemia, finger clubbing or oedema which do not easily fit into any one system or which relate to a number of systems.

The other physical signs are conventionally documented according to body systems as follows:

- General features
- Cardiovascular system (CVS)
- Respiratory system (RS)
- Alimentary system (AS)
- Central nervous system (CNS)
- Locomotor system

However, from a practical point of view the clinical examination of the patient takes place from 'head to toe', rather than 'system by system'. This will minimise the degree of patient discomfort by enabling the signs of different systems which are in the same anatomical area to be demonstrated at the same time. For example, the groin contains the femoral artery (cardiovascular system), lymph nodes (general) and the possibility of hernia (abdominal system) and these can all be assessed at the same time.

In the chapters which follow, each system is considered separately. This may involve some repetition but it is essential that you are able to examine any of the systems in isolation if necessary. However, it is also important that you are able to perform a clinical examination as a whole (from 'top to toe') and the following scheme is given as a guideline:

Begin with the patient lying comfortably in bed resting on pillows at an angle of about 45°. The upper and lower parts should each be covered with blanket so that one may be removed in turn to expose the upper or lower body leaving the other well clad. By convention the examiner stands to the right of the patient and uses his right hand for examination. This may pose problems for the left-handed examiner and if at all possible he* should master all the techniques of examination using his* right hand. Very frequently examination couches in the out-patient department are placed against a wall such that approach from the left side is impossible and the layout of hospital wards is designed with the right-handed person in mind.

In general, you should always compare like with like (usually left and right) and if there is an obvious abnormality you should start by examining the apparently normal side first. Continue to talk while the examination is in progress, possibly exploring some aspects of the history in more detail. Make a general assessment from the foot of the bed and note any obvious abnormalities of position, hair, facies, breathlessness, etc.

Examine the hands and nails, compare radial and brachial pulses on the two sides. Feel for epitrochlear gland enlargement and note any joint abnormalities.

Examine the head and neck to include jugular veins, carotid arteries, oral cavity (mucous membranes, tongue, teeth), thyroid, trachea and neck lymph nodes. The eyes should be examined for any obvious abnormality such as jaundice or anaemia, and assessment of neurological function of the eyes and other cranial nerves may be performed at this stage or at the end of the examination if it is likely that there will be neurological abnormality.

Next expose the chest, but make sure that the abdomen and legs remain covered. Examine the cardiac and respiratory systems, sitting the patient up only once so that posterior chest, spine, renal angles and sacral area can be examined at the same time. Then examine the breasts and axillae, note any obvious neuromuscular problems of the upper limbs, assess the tendon reflexes, and allow the patient to cover the upper half.

Then examine the abdomen (keeping the genital region covered), the groins for lymphadenopathy and the femoral pulse and check the hernial orifices. Look for delay between radial and femoral pulses (particularly if hypertension is the problem) and examine the external genitalia.

The lower limbs are now exposed, keeping the genital region and abdomen covered. Note any abnormalities of the skin, joints and pulses. Finally, examine for wasting, power, tone, reflexes, plantar responses and (where appropriate) sensation.

Finally take the blood pressure – the patient will be relatively relaxed after completion of the examination – and perform a rectal examination.

If the problem is likely to be neurological then a more formal examination of the nervous system is appropriate and this is best conducted as a complete 'system' even if it means going over some of the ground already covered.

The physical examination has several objectives:

- To determine or look for a physical cause for the patient's symptoms and, if possible, assess its nature, extent and severity. Abnormalities that are found on physical examination may confirm a diagnosis made from the history.
- To obtain objective evidence of apparent normality as well as abnormality in various parts of the body.
- To screen for abnormalities of which the patient may be unaware and which may be unrelated to the presenting condition such as hypertension or rectal carcinoma.

Failing to demonstrate important signs or abnormalities is minimised by conducting the examination methodically. The conventional order is:

- Inspection
- Palpation

- Percussion
- Auscultation

Inspection

This means looking for (rather than looking at) and implies observation with particular features in mind. It is, therefore, important to know what you are looking for in both the normal and abnormal state.

Palpation

This is the use of touch to determine the characteristics of normal and abnormal areas of the body. The flat of the hand is usually used with the pulps of the fingers being the most sensitive and gentle. Palpation is used to assess tenderness, pulsatility, size and mobility of a mass.

Fluctuation may be determined by placing the second and third fingers of each hand at right angles on either side of the mass. Movement in more than one direction (i.e. fluctuation) suggests that the mass contains fluid that is not under tension (such as pus in an abscess).

Percussion

This is an important technique that must be mastered. It will help to distinguish between solid, gas and fluid and considerably improves the diagnostic accuracy of physical examination.

The left hand is placed with the fingers spread slightly, so that the second phalanx of the middle finger is firmly applied to the area to be percussed. The right middle finger then strikes the phalanx at right angles to produce a hammer effect with all the movement of the right hand coming from the wrist (see Fig 2.).

The percussion note is assessed by the pitch of the noise produced and also by the vibration felt by the middle finger of the left hand. It is, therefore, not necessary (and usually counterproductive) to produce a loud sound by forceful percussion, which may be uncomfortable to the patient.

The percussion note is documented as follows:

- Resonant – tissue containing air, e.g. normal lung
- Dull – solid organ, e.g. liver
- Tympanitic – hollow air-containing structure, e.g. stomach
- Hyper-resonant – lung with decreased density, e.g. emphysema or pneumothorax
- Flat – percussion over a large muscle mass e.g. thigh

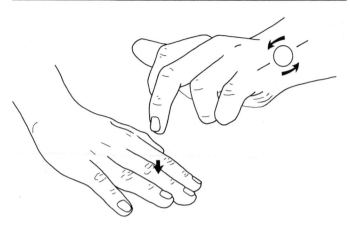

Fig. 2.   Percussion technique.

Percussion should be performed from resonant areas to dull with the left finger parallel to the edge of the structure to be examined and the percussion note of similar structures on two sides compared. Therefore, when percussing the posterior chest you should go from left to right comparing the note at the same level.

Auscultation

Auscultation usually involves listening with the stethoscope, an instrument that conducts sounds to the listening ears. The ear pieces should be inserted into the ears correctly (pointing forwards) and the bell or diaphragm applied firmly to the skin so as to form an air-tight seal. In general the bell of the stethoscope is better for detecting low pitched sounds and the diaphragm for higher, but the bell may be used when the diaphragm is picking up unwanted sounds (such as auscultation over a hairy chest). The diaphragm should be warmed before use, the bell usually has a rubber ring. The stethoscope is frequently used to listen for the sound of turbulent flow in the vascular system. When this occurs in the heart the noise is called a murmur, and when the turbulence is in blood vessels the term is bruit. The absence of sound may be important as in the 'silent abdomen' of peritonitis.

It is important to be able to measure the enlargement or displacement of organs and dimensions of a lump or mass. A tape measure is very valuable but if you measure the length and width of your index finger you will have a readily available measure without recourse on each occasion to the use of a tape measure. Inaccurate documentation (e.g. 'two fingerbreadths enlarged') can be replaced easily by an objective measurement in centimeters.

Details of the examination are recorded in the case notes system by system. You will not be able to write notes as you perform the clinical examination so it is important to note mentally any abnormality as you go along, and at the end assume that the rest of the systematic examination was normal. This is only possible if you have a 'template' of clinical examination to work from and this is why it is essential that you have a standard routine to follow. You will, of course have to remember such details as the pulse rate and blood pressure.

Even if the clinical examination is entirely normal there are certain important (normal) details which should be recorded in the notes. These form the basis for the 'Minimal statement of the examination of a system' which are given at the end of each section, and should be documented in every case, even if there are no morbid signs.

*The **examination of any lump or mass** can be used to illustrate the conventional order of examination as follows:*

- *Inspection*
  Anatomical location
  Colour
  Movement (with respiration for example)
  Pulsation
  Changes in the overlying skin
    – Peau d'orange *due to dermal oedema*
    – *Erythema due to inflammation or infection*
  Transillumination
    – *A bright light shone through the mass will distinguish whether it is fluid- or air-filled or solid.*

- *Palpation*
  Situation with regard to other structures
    – *Within skin or muscle, or in the thyroid gland*
    – *Attachment to structures, mobility*
  Shape and size
  Consistency including fluctuation
  Pulsation – Whether transmitted or expansile?
        – *Can it be emptied of its contents? (e.g. hernia)*

- *Percussion*
  e.g. Stony dull percussion note suggests fluid-filled mass such as urinary bladder

- *Auscultation*
  Arterial or venous bruits
  Bowel sounds

2 General examination

Document:

> *Height, weight*
> *Temperature*
> *Pulse rate*
> *Respiration rate*
> *Blood pressure*

Observe:

General condition	–	*well/ill*
		comfortable/in pain
		breathless
Physical appearance	–	*thin, fat, big frame, muscular*
		biological age
Position in bed	–	*propped up*
		lying flat comfortably
		restless
Mental state	–	*alert, drowsy, confused, co-operative*
Nutrition	–	*wasted, dehydrated, recent weight loss*
Skin	–	*pallor, cyanosis, jaundice*
		pigmentation, rashes, striae
		spider naevi.
Mucous membranes	–	*pallor, pigmentation*
Hands	–	*palmar erythema*
		Dupuytren's contracture
Nails	–	*clubbing, koilonychia*
		splinter haemorrhages, pitting
Hair	–	*texture*
		alopecia, hirsutism
Fetor	–	*ketones, alcohol*
		hepatic and uraemic

Eyes	–	*colour of sclerae, exophthalmos*
Neck	–	*lymph nodes, venous engorgement*
		pulsation or tumours

Thyroid gland
Breasts

First impressions of your patient are very important and with practice and experience you may be able to make a 'spot diagnosis' (such as acromegaly, dystrophia myotonica or peritonitis) based on the patient's appearance and behaviour. The record of the general examination should be a word-picture of the patient's general condition and include a statement about certain abnormalities which are sought in every case. It is not, therefore, limited to the initial observations of the patient.

Height, weight, nutrition

The **Body Mass Index** (BMI – Quetelet's Index) is most commonly used to measure obesity and is derived from the formula:

Weight (kg)/Height $(M)^2$

The definition of obesity using BMI is shown in the table below.

BMI	Grade	Description
20–25	0	Ideal weight range
25–30	1	Overweight
30–40	2	Moderately obese
> 40	3	Grossly obese

Note the distribution of obesity, because an increase in abdominal girth (particularly in men) is associated with an increased risk of cardiovascular disease, whereas the relationship is less strong when just body weight and not its distribution is taken into account. Objective assessment of weight distribution may be made by measuring the waist circumference and comparing it with the circumference at the hips – the waist–hip ratio, which should not significantly exceed unity in men.

The height and weight of children (from birth to 19 years old) can be plotted using the Tanner-Whitehouse Standard Chart. This allows the height and weight to be expressed as a percentile in comparison with the normal population of a given age. In addition, growth velocity can be calculated if measurements are taken over a 1 year period.

There are many causes of weight loss, which when extreme is called cachexia (often due to malignancy).

Dehydration may be determined initially by lack of elasticity of the skin which is tested by gently pinching up a small fold of skin over the anterior chest wall between finger and thumb and noting that it will not quickly resume its normal contour. However, the elderly often have inelastic skin in the absence of dehydration. Dryness of the tongue is often said to be a useful indicator of dehydration but the commonest cause of a dry tongue is not dehydration but mouth breathing. A more accurate clinical assessment of dehydration may be obtained by noting that the jugular venous pressure is not visible (even when the patient is lying flat and pressure is applied to the epigastrium) and lack of distension of the veins on the hands (or the head of a baby).

Temperature

This is measured in degrees Celsius (°C) using a mercury thermometer placed under the patient's tongue (oral temperature). If the patient is unable to tolerate the thermometer under his* tongue because of restlessness or jaw clenching then it may be placed in the axilla (or in the fold of the groin in children), where the recorded temperature is half a degree lower than in the mouth. When hypothermia is suspected a low-reading thermometer (with a blue bulb) is placed in the rectum, where the recording is the same as that in the mouth.

The normal temperature varies between 36.5°C and 37.2°C. There is a diurnal variation, with temperature highest at around 10 p.m. and lowest at 2 a.m. Heat is lost by sweating and it is not uncommon to have 'night sweats' because of the normal temperature fall in the early hours of the morning. There is also a menstrual variation in women with the temperature highest at the time of ovulation (a temperature chart may help to identify the time of ovulation).

Hypothermia is defined as a temperature below 35°C and may be due in young people to acute exposure, and in the elderly or infirm to gradual loss of body temperature in association with conditions such as stroke and immobility.

Fever is a temperature above 37.2°C. Pyrogens (which may be endogenous or exogenous) act on the hypothalamic temperature regulating centre probably via prostaglandins to cause a rise in temperature. This is achieved by reducing peripheral blood flow which reduces heat loss, and shivering which generates heat. If the temperature rise is sudden the patient feels very cold and is shivering violently – a rigor. When the higher temperature has been achieved the patient feels burningly hot (pyrexia) and often has a headache.

There are three patterns of fever which were thought to have important diagnostic value:

- Continued fever does not fluctuate by more than 1°C and does not fall to within the normal range. Typhoid fever is a good example.
- Remittent fever fluctuates by more than 2°C but does not reach normal. This is also called hectic or swinging pyrexia and suggests a collection of pus (gall bladder, kidney or subphrenic abscess).
- Intermittent fever is present for only a few hours during the 24 h period and suggests malaria or malignancy.

However, many infections are modified early in their course by antibiotics and these 'classic' patterns lose their diagnostic value.

The pulse rate increases by about 10 beats per minute with each 1°C rise in body temperature.

Observation

Attitude is the term used to describe the position that the patient adopts. He* may be sitting upright and leaning forwards due to breathlessness, pericarditis or pancreatic pain; lying flat and very still due to peritonitis; moving about restlessly trying to find a comfortable position with colic; or in an awkward position due to general or focal weakness.

The chronological age will be apparent from the recorded date of birth but many patients look much older (or sometimes younger) than their years (**biological age**). A long history of cigarette smoking may lead to 'smoker's face' where the skin is thickened, lined and sallow giving the appearance of advanced biological age. These changes may be associated with similar degenerative change internally with an increased incidence of coronary artery disease and emphysema. Severe weight loss from any cause may add to the appearance of premature aging.

Skin

Abnormality of the skin may be noted in primary dermatological conditions (such as psoriasis and eczema) as well as in systemic illness. In addition, conditions like psoriasis frequently have systemic effects. It is, therefore, very important to examine the skin carefully. However, only a few of the more common disorders which point to systemic disease will be discussed here.

Pallor suggests anaemia but may be seen in any acute painful illness. The pallor of anaemia is best observed in the mucous membrane of the mouth and in the conjunctiva and nail bed (in the absence of coloured nail varnish). Anaemia is notoriously difficult to detect and quantify clinically because the skin may be tanned or weather-beaten; the conjuctivae may look red due to inflammation; and the elderly often look pale. The only sure way to detect anaemia is to measure the haemoglobin concentration of the blood.

Spider naevi are very characteristic abnormalities of cutaneous arterioles, which may indicate liver cirrhosis. The centre of the 'spider' is a dilated arteriole and the 'legs' are due to small blood vessels radiating from the centre. Compression of the central arteriole (with a pin head or glass slide) will cause blanching. Spider naevi occur in the distribution of the superior vena cava (for reasons that are not known). Women (particularly those who are pregnant or taking an oral contraceptive pill) are allowed up to three spiders (men none) and any more are considered to be of pathological significance.

Erythema ab igne is brown discolouration of the skin which has a reticular pattern and is due to chronic damage by heat to the vascular arcades of the dermis and deposition of haemosiderin in the skin. This pattern is commonly seen on the shins of elderly ladies (who wear stockings rather than trousers) who sit in front of a fire to keep warm. However, when observed elsewhere erythema ab igne may have diagnostic significance as patients will tend to try to alleviate chronic pain by applying a heat pad or hot water bottle over the site of the pain. Thus, erythema ab igne noted in the skin of the right upper abdominal quadrant may suggest chronic cholecystitis. A similar pattern of skin discolouration (*livedo reticularis*) is seen in vasculitis.

Cyanosis describes the blue appearance of mucous membranes, or skin, due to the presence of more than (approximately) 5 g/100 ml deoxygenated haemoglobin in the circulation (arterial oxygen saturation below about 80%). It may be central or peripheral.

● Central cyanosis occurs when deoxygenated blood mixes with oxygenated 'arterial' blood in the heart, great vessels or lungs. Causes include right-to-left cardiac shunts (often congenital – cyanotic congenital heart disease); arterio-venous shunts in the lungs; and severe hypoxic lung disease. Cyanosis is more obvious when there is an increase of haemoglobin and red cells in the circulation (polycythaemia). The tongue is the best place to look for central cyanosis because it is always well perfused. Cyanosis detected in the hands or nails is central if the hands are warm.

● Peripheral cyanosis occurs when local circulation is impaired and there is greater extraction of oxygen from the haemoglobin by the tissues. The cyanosis is seen in the peripheral circulation such as hands and feet and these are usually cold. Poor peripheral circulation may be confirmed by assessing the return of capillary flow to the nail bed following pressure on the distal nail plate.

Jaundice is the yellow appearance of the sclerae, mucous membranes and skin caused by an increase in plasma bilirubin concentration, which has to be raised 3 times above the normal before the jaundice is clinically apparent. Jaundice is most reliably detected in the sclerae because yellow skin may be a racial phenomenon or due to staining from drugs (e.g. mepacrin). However, yellow staining of the sclerae is due only to bilirubin (although the elderly tend to have a rather yellow appearance to the sclerae). There may also be a difference in colour between the hard and the soft palate, the latter assuming an orange rather than the usual pink colour in the presence of jaundice.

Where the cause of jaundice is haemolysis (drug-induced or haemoglobinopathies, for example) the jaundice is pale yellow. In chronic obstructive jaundice (such as in primary biliary cirrhosis) the jaundice deepens to a brownish-green colour and is associated with pruritus (irritation/itching of the skin caused by an increase in circulating bile salts), pale stools and dark urine.

Hands

Palmar erythema is the red colour of the skin of the hands (particularly affecting the thenar and hypothenar eminences) that occurs in liver cirrhosis. It may be seen in normal persons and is a poor clinical sign.

Dupuytren's contracture is a fibrotic process affecting the palmar fascia, which leads to puckering of the overlying skin and fixed flexion of the fingers related to the involved fascia (usually the ring and little fingers). The contracture and flexion may be obvious on inspection but lesser degrees can be identified by feeling the palm transversely and noting the thickening. It is said that there is an association with alcoholic cirrhosis, but this is not reliable. Dupuytren's contracture is more frequent with increasing age, particularly in men and usually there is no significant association with any underlying condition. However, if the contractures affect predominantly the fascia of the middle fingers then there is an association with diabetes (diabetic cheiro-arthropathy).

Nails

Clubbing (see Fig. 3) was first described by Hippocrates and its pathogenesis is still unclear. However, it is likely that there is a neurocirculatory component because the constant feature of clubbing

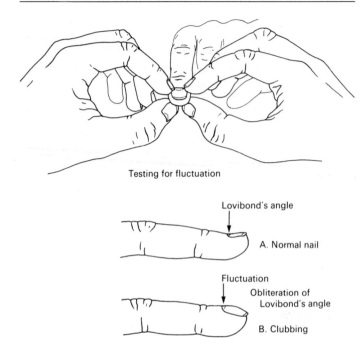

Testing for fluctuation

A. Normal nail — Lovibond's angle

B. Clubbing — Fluctuation, Obliteration of Lovibond's angle

Fig. 3.   Clubbing of the nails.

(and the first physical sign) is an increase in the vascularity of the distal fingers and consequently an increased sponginess of the nail bed. This may be demonstrated by rocking the distal end of the nail and observing excessive movement of the proximal end, or by exerting pressure over the proximal nail plate and feeling fluctuation. As clubbing progresses the swollen tissues lift the proximal nail to obliterate and then reverse the angle between the nail fold and the nail plate. There is then increased curvature of the nails in both longitudinal and lateral axes and, finally, the ends of the fingers become bulbous, like drum sticks.

Clubbing tends to affect the index finger first and it is this finger that should be examined. If bulbous enlargement is not obvious, test for proximal fluctuation ('floating nail') and then observe the finger from the lateral aspect to assess the nailfold/nail-plate angle (Lovibond's angle) which should normally be less than 180°.

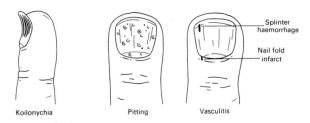

Fig. 4.   Some appearances of the nails.

Clubbing may be congenital and familial, but acquired clubbing is a very valuable sign of underlying disorders the commonest of which are as follows:

- Respiratory system
  Bronchial carcinoma
  Chronic intrathoracic sepsis – empyema, lung abscess, bronchiectasis
  Pulmonary fibrosis – fibrosing alveolitis

- Cardiovascular system
  Cyanotic congenital heart disease
  Infective endocarditis

- Gastrointestinal system
  Inflammatory bowel disease – ulcerative colitis, Crohn's disease
  Cirrhosis of the liver
  Malabsorption

Chronic bronchitis is NOT a cause of clubbing and carcinoma should be suspected.

Koilonychia (Fig. 4) refers to brittle nails with characteristic spoon shape which will hold a globule of water and which suggest chronic iron deficiency anaemia.

Splinter haemorrhages (Fig. 4) are longitudinal dark lines seen under the nail plate and are due to small haemorrhages from vasculitis. They appear as 'splinters' because the nail bed is thrown into a series of longitudinal ridges and the haemorrhage tracks along these ridges. The splinter haemorrhages may be better observed by illuminating the nail bed with a torch pressed against the tip of the pulp of the finger.

The commonest cause of splinter haemorrhages of the finger nails is recurrent minor trauma. Therefore, to confirm their pathological significance examine the toe nails for splinter haemorrhages and also the conjunctivae where 'blot' haemorrhages suggest vasculitis.

Thick, yellow, **pitted** nails (Fig. 4) are characteristic of the changes associated with psoriasis. Nail involvement occurs in approximately half of patients with psoriasis, particularly in those with arthropathy.

White nails (**leuconychia**) are seen in states of low serum albumen such as cirrhosis of the liver and nephrotic syndrome, but may also be congenital.

Fetor

This is the term given to the smell of the breath and implies more than the potential social problem of halitosis. Foul smelling breath may be due to infections of the mouth (including gums and teeth), lung abscess (particularly when there is anaerobic infection) and the presence of altered blood in the stomach. In addition, there may be particular smells which reflect metabolic abnormality such as the sweet aroma (fermenting hay or mice) of liver failure, the uriniferous smell of renal failure, and the 'pear-drop' smell of ketones in diabetic keto-acidosis. The smell of alcohol on the breath is often very useful in diagnosis.

2.1   Examination of the thyroid gland

- *Inspection*
  The normal thyroid gland is not obvious on inspection. Have the patient sit in front of you with neck exposed and ask him* to swallow (give him* a glass of water if necessary). The thyroid gland moves with the thyroid cartilage (Adam's apple) on swallowing.

- *Palpation*
  Feel the thyroid gland with the fingers of both hands gently from the front and again from behind with the patient swallowing. Assess the size of the gland, its consistency, whether it is smooth or nodular and whether there is any associated lymph node enlargement.

- *Auscultation*
  Listen with the stethoscope over both lobes for a bruit which suggests increased vascularity of a toxic thyroid gland.

2.2 Examination of the lymphatic system

Examine the neck for enlarged lymph nodes to include the preauricular, post-auricular, submental, submandibular, superficial and deep cervical, occipital and subclavian regions. Most of these nodes are best palpated from behind with the patient sitting.

Examine epitrochlear, axillary and groin regions.

Look for enlargement of veins at the root of the neck or front of the chest which may suggest mediastinal glandular enlargement. The para-aortic glands should be carefully palpated when examining the abdomen.

Describe the location and size of any enlarged nodes and also their consistency (hard, firm, rubbery).

The examination of the lymphatic system is completed by excluding enlargement of the spleen.

Lymphoid tissue (including the spleen) tends to atrophy with age and younger persons will normally have some enlarged lymph nodes, particularly submandibular (due to recurrent infection of the tonsils) and in the groins (small 'shotty' nodes from minor infection of the toes). Axillary nodes may be palpable in manual workers who frequently traumatise their hands and arms.

Metastatic carcinoma tends to cause hard lymph node enlargement; infection leads to soft, tender enlargement; and lymphoma causes massive, rubbery, firm nodes which form a confluent mass. An increasingly frequent cause of generalised lymphadenopathy is human immuno deficiency virus (HIV) disease (Persistent generalised lymphadenopathy – PGL).

A hard gland in the left supraclavicular fossa (Virchow's node) suggests carcinoma of the stomach. Epitrochlear glands tend to be enlarged in sarcoidosis and syphilis and also in generalised viral infection such as glandular fever.

Para-aortic and other retroperitoneal glands are very difficult to detect clinically, but enlargement is very important in conditions such as testicular tumour and lymphoma. Abdominal ultrasound in slim subjects and computed tomography in the more obese subjects (FAT = CAT) are the investigations of choice to detect these glands.

2.3 Examination of the breast

One pair of breasts develops in the pectoral region from the milk line which extends from the axillae to the inguinal region. Accessory breasts (usually just the nipple) may occur anywhere along this line (but most commonly just below the normal breast) and are of no clinical significance.

The male breast

Gynaecomastia is enlargement of the male breast and is due to an excess of oestrogen compared with testosterone. It occurs frequently in the elderly (declining levels of testosterone) and in obese subjects (increased formation of oestrogens in adipose tissue) in whom it is important to distinguish true retroareolar glandular tissue from fat.

When gynaecomastia is painful or rapidly enlarging a search must be made for the source of oestrogen over-production such as the testis (teratoma) and adrenal gland. Cirrhosis of the liver causes gynaecomastia (and spider naevi and testicular atrophy) because there is reduced hepatic metabolism of normal oestrogens.

The female breast

For documentation and descriptive purposes the breast is divided into four quadrants by a horizontal and a vertical line passing through the nipple (upper/outer, lower/medial etc.).

- *Inspection of the female breast*
  Ask the patient to sit facing you and to remove her gown to the waist. With her hands by her side note:
  Shape, symmetry, contour and obvious mass
  Erythema, peau d'orange or dimpling of the skin
  Nipple retraction, fissuring, scaling or redness
  Then ask the patient to press her hands against her hips to tense the pectoral muscles which may accentuate abnormality of contour or skin dimpling if there is a mass attached to muscle.

- *Palpation of the female breast*
  Now ask the patient to lie on her back with one hand (right hand for right breast and vice versa) under her head to spread out the breast tissue evenly over the chest wall. Gently palpate the four quadrants with the flat of the hand and finger tips and note the characteristics of any mass which is felt.
  Examine the axillary lymph nodes.
  If the complaint is of nipple discharge it is probably best to ask the woman to express the discharge from the nipple herself.

Breast cancer is the most common malignant disease in women and perhaps one woman in ten (in UK and USA) will be affected at some time during her life. There is a tendency for breast cancer to be familial with first-degree relatives of a woman with pre-menopausal breast cancer having three times the risk of developing the disease when compared with the general population, but if the woman has cancer in both breasts the risk to her first-degree relatives is nearly ten times. Most breast cancers are detected as painless lumps by either the patient (who is encouraged to self-examine her breasts), or her doctor during a routine physical examination. Routine examination of the breast is important, particularly in women with a positive family history as the sooner the diagnosis is made the better is the prognosis. Breast screening with mammography is becoming an increasingly common procedure.

2.4 Minimal statement of the general examination

Healthy looking, well nourished
No jaundice, anaemia, cyanosis, clubbing (JACC°)
Thyroid not enlarged (Thyroid°)
No lymphadenopathy (LN°)
Breasts normal

3 Examination of the cardiovascular system

3.1 General

Note

Evidence of generalised disease
Smoker's face, ear-lobe crease
Attitude – able to lie flat, sitting upright
Shortness of breath
Cyanosis
Clubbing, splinter haemorrhages
Dependent oedema
    legs, sacrum
    describe the degree of pitting, its distribution
    associated varicose veins

Stigmata of hyperlipidaemia
  corneal arcus
  xanthelasmata
  tendon xanthomata
Peripheral perfusion
Varicose veins and evidence of venous insufficiency, ulceration
Presence of crackles at lung bases
Tender enlargement of the liver

Generalised disease

This may affect the cardiovascular system as follows:

- Down's syndrome – congenital heart disease such as atrio-septal defect, and ventriculo-septal defect with mitral regurgitation.
- Turner's syndrome – coarctation of the aorta.
- Thyrotoxicosis – atrial fibrillation and heart failure.
- Marfan's syndrome – aortic root dilatation with tendency to dissection and rupture; mitral valve disease.
- Ankylosing spondylitis – mitral and aortic valvular disease.
- Alcoholism – dilated cardiomyopathy.

Pectus excavatum may be a forme fruste of Marfan syndrome and is associated with mitral valve prolapse. The distance between the spine and sternum is reduced resulting in an apparent enlargement of the heart on chest radiograph and functional systolic murmur.

Clinical features that suggest **cardiac failure** include:

Sitting upright, breathless
Peripheral oedema
Crackles at lung bases
Tender, enlarged liver

The presence of an **earlobe crease** is associated with an increased likelihood of coronary artery disease.

Smoker's face is one which appears older than its chronological age, looks gaunt with sunken cheeks. The skin is thickened and sallow with deep creases, particularly around the mouth. This appearance is strongly correlated with heavy tobacco use but may also be seen in the very elderly and those chronically exposed to the weather.

Dependent oedema

When the pressure in the peripheral veins is high (due to raised right atrial pressure in heart failure, or to venous obstruction from thrombo-

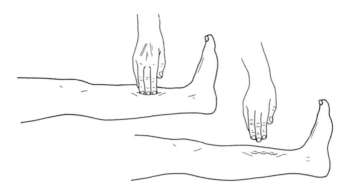

Fig. 5. Pitting oedema.

sis); or when the oncotic pressure of the plasma is reduced (in states of
low serum albumen); or when the lymphatic drainage is reduced, then
fluid may accumulate in the interstitial space and cause oedema. Its
distribution will depend on gravity, such that in ambulant patients (or
those sitting with their legs dependent) the fluid will collect in the legs
and in those who are confined to bed it will tend to accumulate over the
lower back and sacrum. When oedema is extensive it will be distributed
from the feet to the abdominal wall.

*The characteristic feature of **pitting oedema** is that when the
skin is pressed, an indentation will remain which can be seen and
felt. Small amounts are best demonstrated by pressing gently for
about 30 s with the thumb or three fingers over the shin and
feeling the indentation which is left when the pressure is removed
(see Fig. 5).*

Oedema which does not pit is described as 'brawny' and is due to
organisation of the oedema fluid in the interstitial space. This is seen in
chronic venous oedema and also in lymphatic obstruction.

Oedema is frequently seen in association with varicose veins and
may be due to previous venous thrombosis. There is often brown
pigmentation of the skin (due to haemosiderin) and fibrosis of the
subcutaneous tissues (lipodermatosclerosis) in a 'gaiter' distribution
round the lower third of the leg with a tendency to ulcer formation
particularly on the medial side. The commonest cause of peripheral
oedema is immobility often in association with obesity.

Stigmata of hyperlipidaemia

Corneal arcus is a grey-white ring at the periphery of the cornea. It may be a normal finding in older persons (hence the misleading term *arcus senilis*) but if it is very obvious or noted in younger patients then it is important to consider hypercholesterolaemia as a cause.

Xanthoma is a collection of lipid presenting as a painless lump often associated with the tendons of the hand or heel and extensor surfaces, such as the elbow. A similar collection of lipid may occur in the skin where it appears as a yellow plaque, particularly of the eyelids when it is termed **xanthelasma**. These lipid collections have a strong association with abnormal lipid metabolism and are important to note in the clinical evaluation of familial hyperlipidaemia.

Peripheral perfusion

Perfusion of the limbs may be clinically assessed by noting whether they are warm or cold; whether there is normal distribution of hair; whether the nails and skin are normal; and whether the normal pink colour rapidly returns to the nail bed when pressure on the nail is withdrawn.

3.2   Arterial pulse

Note

> *Rate and rhythm (from palpation of radial pulse)*
> *Character (from palpation of brachial or carotid arteries)*
> *Peripheral pulses (temporal, carotid, brachial, radial, femoral, popliteal, dorsalis pedis, posterior tibial)*

Rate

The normal range is by convention between 60–90 beats per min. If regular the pulse rate may be counted over either 10 or 15 s (and multiplied by either 6 or 4) but if irregular 30 s is recommended. A very accurate measurement of pulse rate is not necessary.

Bradycardia is a pulse rate below 60 bpm and may be observed in:

Trained athletes, normal sleep
Hypothyroidism
Hypothermia
Raised intracranial pressure
Treatment with drugs such as beta-blockers, digoxin, diltiazem
Heart block

Tachycardia is a pulse rate above 90 bpm and may be observed in:

Exercise, anxiety
Fever
Hyperthyroidism
Shock due to blood loss or heart failure
Treatment with drugs such as nifedipine, theophylline
Atrial or ventricular tachycardias

Rhythm

The rhythm may be:

- Regular in which case normal sinus rhythm is assumed
- Regularly irregular where every second, third or fourth beat is regularly 'dropped'
- Irregularly irregular due either to atrial fibrillation or multiple ectopic beats
- Accelerating on inspiration and slowing on expiration (sinus arr-hythmia) – a common normal finding particularly in children
- Regular with occasional 'dropped' beats (ectopic beats). The patient describes a missed beat followed by an exaggerated beat.

Atrial fibrillation (AF) may be distinguished clinically from multiple ectopic beats by:

- Absence of 'a'-wave in jugular venous pulse
- Tendency for ectopic beats to disappear with exercise (sitting up and down), whereas atrial fibrillation becomes more chaotic

However, the definitive diagnosis can only be made using the electrocardiogram.

The pulse deficit at the wrist (the difference between the pulse rate determined at the cardiac apex and that measured at the wrist) is not helpful in the diagnosis of atrial fibrillation. The pulse will be 'dropped' at the wrist if cardiac contraction occurs when the left ventricle is partially empty of blood. Filling of the ventricle takes place in diastole and any cardiac rhythm which causes a short diastolic filling time will lead to apical-radial pulse deficit.

Character

The character of the pulse is best assessed by palpation of the carotid arteries, which reflect the activity of the left ventricle modified as little as possible by factors such as arterial wall compliance which may occur in the more distal pulses. The carotid arteries should be palpated gently (particularly in the elderly) and one at a time with the thumb or three fingers. It is the waveform that is felt and it is incorrect to use the term 'volume' (although everyone will know what you mean!).

The following pulse characteristics are recognised:

- Normal
- Slow rising upstroke – aortic stenosis
- Rapid upstroke and downstroke (collapsing) – aortic regurgitation, arterio-venous fistula, hyperdynamic circulation
- Small amplitude (volume) – measured as the pulse pressure and found in low output states e.g. heart failure, shock; and severe mitral stenosis
- *Pulsus paradoxus* – a reduction in systolic blood pressure by more than 10 mmHg on inspiration and seen in constrictive pericarditis or severe asthma

Peripheral pulses

A pulse may be felt at any site where an artery is superficial and can be compressed against a firm structure such as bone. For example the carotid pulse is felt by compressing the carotid artery posteriorly against one of the cervical vertebral transverse processes. It is best to feel the pulses with two or three finger tips (index, middle and ring) so that the waveform can be appreciated. The thumb may be used to palpate large arteries (brachial and carotid) but otherwise should not be used as it tends to be pulsatile itself and this may interfere with palpation of smaller arteries.

Compare the pulses on the two sides and record whether equal, diminished or absent and the presence of a bruit. The following pulses (Fig. 6) should be identified:

- *Superficial temporals are felt in front of the upper border of the ear and run upwards and medially over the forehead.*
- *Carotids (the common or external carotid artery) can be felt by pressing posteriorly into the neck between the larynx and sternomastoid. The arteries should be felt one at a time with particular care being taken in the elderly, and a pulse may be felt even if the artery is thrombosed. Listen for a bruit.*
- *Brachial arteries can be felt on the medial side of the antecubital fossa.*
- *Radial arteries are felt by pressing over the radial styloid at the level of the watch strap.*

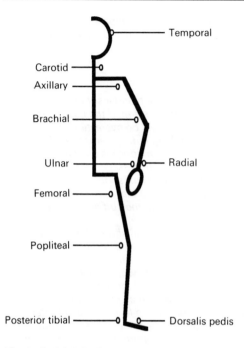

Fig. 6.   Peripheral pulses.

- *Femoral arteries are felt just below the inguinal ligament half way between the superior anterior iliac spine and the symphysis pubis. Listen for a bruit.*
- *Popliteal arteries are often difficult to feel even in health. Exert firm pressure in the popliteal fossa in the mid-line with the fingers of both hands with the knee relaxed at about 45°.*
- *Posterior tibial pulses are felt behind and below the medial malleolus.*
- *Dorsalis pedis pulses are felt over the dorsum of the foot lateral to the tendon of tibialis anterior and the prominence caused by the second cuneiform bone.*

Inequality of the upper limb pulses suggests coarctation or dissection of the aorta.

The leg pulses are delayed and weak compared with the radial pulse (radio-femoral delay) in coarctation and dissection of the aorta.

3.3   Measurement of blood pressure

The width and length of the inflatable bladder should be appropriate for the size of the patient's arm. If the bladder is too short or narrow the blood pressure will be overestimated. Therefore, ensure that a wide or long cuff ('alternative adult' – bladder 13–15 cm wide and 30–35 cm long) is used for an average sized arm and larger may be necessary for an obese or very muscular arm. Similarly a smaller cuff should be used for children. The patient should be warned that minor discomfort may be experienced by the inflation of the cuff and that several readings may be necessary.

The patient may be sitting or lying, and should be warm and relaxed having spent 3 min in the chosen position. Standing blood pressure should be recorded after 1 min of assuming the upright position, particularly in patients with diabetes and those taking anti-hypertensive medication and the elderly when a postural fall in systolic blood pressure may be anticipated. The patient's arm should be horizontal at the level of the mid-sternum (dependency of the arm below the heart increases the blood pressure by about 10 mmHg) and supported so that there is no isometric muscle contraction (which will also raise the blood pressure).

Tight clothing should be removed from the arm and the centre of the bladder (often marked) applied over the brachial artery (determined by palpation medial to the biceps tendon) so that the lower end of the cuff is about 2 cm above the antecubital fossa. The mercury column should be vertical and at eye level (stand mounted manometers are recommended). The cuff should be inflated until the brachial artery pulse disappears and then deflated slowly until the systolic blood pressure is determined by palpation (the pressure at which the pulse is first felt). The patient may be aware of this return of blood flow.

The stethoscope is applied to the brachial artery in the antecubital fossa and the cuff inflated to about 30 mmHg above the previously estimated systolic blood pressure. The pressure is reduced at about 2 mmHg per heart beat until clear tapping sounds first appear for two consecutive heart beats. This is the

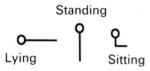

Standing

Lying   Sitting

Fig. 7.   Symbols to note the position of the patient.

systolic blood pressure (Karotkoff sound I). The point where the sounds muffle is Karotkoff sound IV and where they finally disappear is sound V.

Record systolic blood pressure and diastolic blood pressure phase V, unless this is difficult to identify, in which case use phase IV.

Note which arm was used for recording the blood pressure and the position of the patient (Fig. 7)

Lying (. . . .)
Sitting (. . . .)
Standing (. . . .).

The blood pressure should be recorded twice within about 3 min and the average value of systolic and diastolic pressures be recorded.

In the initial assessment of hypertension the blood pressure should be recorded in both arms. If relevant note whether systolic blood pressure varies with respiration. Where atrial fibrillation is present take an average of several recordings.

Important clinical decisions are made on the basis of blood pressure readings so it is vital that good technique is used to ensure accurate measurement and that the equipment (preferably a mercury sphygmomanometer) is in good working order.

Blood pressure varies during the 24 h day depending on activity (rather than having an intrinsic circadian rhythm) being highest when waking and lowest in the early hours of the morning. It is lower in hot weather and during the summer (irrespective of the prevailing temperature) and tends to rise with age.

Both systolic and diastolic blood pressure are distributed continuously within the population but 160/90 mmHg is taken as the upper limit of 'normal' (WHO).

Hypertension is defined as follows (WHO/International Society of Hypertension):

Definition	Diastolic BP (mmHg)	Systolic BP (mmHg)
● Borderline	90–94	140–160
● Mild	95–104	161–180
● Moderate	105–114	> 180
● Severe	> 115	
● Malignant	> 140	

Isolated systolic hypertension is defined as systolic blood pressure greater than 160 mmHg and diastolic blood pressure less than 90 mmHg.

Blood pressure recordings should be repeated at least three times during a 4 week period before the above definitions are applied.

Hypertension is said to be 'accelerated' (or 'malignant') when the raised diastolic blood pressure (usually greater than 140 mmHg) is associated with papilloedema and a risk of cerebral oedema and acute hypertensive heart failure. This situation is a medical emergency.

3.4   Jugular venous pulse (JVP)

Note

Height of JVP
Character
  Pulsatile or non-pulsatile
  Increase or decrease with inspiration
Waveform
  'a'-wave absent, increased or cannon
  'v'-wave increased.

Height

Because the jugular veins have no valves observation of the venous pulsation in the neck reflects the pressure changes in the right atrium. It is best to observe the internal jugular vein, because the external vein pierces the deep fascia of the neck and may be obstructed, causing the right atrial pressure to be reflected inaccurately. The right atrium lies 5 cm vertically below the manubriosternal angle and as the normal right atrial pressure is about 5 cm of blood this angle may be taken as a reference point, with elevation of the venous pressure above this being abnormal. By convention the patient sits at an angle of 45° to the horizontal, because in this position the distended veins will be just visible above the clavicle if the venous pressure is normal. However, as long as the vertical height above the manubriosternal angle is measured the position of the patient does not matter (the most comfortable being preferable).

The jugular venous pulse is distinguished from the carotid (arterial) pulse because:

- It is not palpable
- It usually has two waves
- An upper vertical height can be determined
- It can be obliterated by pressure above the clavicle
- The waveform is undulating and expansile

If the venous pulse cannot be seen:

- Lie the patient flat or sit him* up
- Ask the patient to perform a Valsalva manoeuvre or press gently on the epigastrium (both will increase the right atrial pressure)
- Trap the lower end of the vein by pressure above the clavicle and watch the vein fill from above

Raised venous pressure indicates increased right atrial pressure due to heart failure, pulmonary embolus or pericardial effusion.

Low venous pressure (when the jugular veins are not visible even on lying flat or with epigastric pressure) indicates hypovolaemia.

Character

Non-pulsatile elevation of venous pressure suggests superior vena caval obstruction. The normal venous pressure falls with inspiration but if it rises (paradoxical or Kussmaul's sign) then constrictive pericarditis or pericardial effusion is likely.

Waveform

Two waves may be identified clinically by observation:

1 The 'a'-wave which is caused by atrial contraction and will be:

- Absent in atrial fibrillation;
- Increased in any condition that causes right atrial overactivity such as pulmonary valve stenosis and pulmonary hypertension;
- Intermittently greatly increased (**cannon wave**) when the right atrium contracts against a closed tricuspid valve as in complete atrioventricular dissociation (heart block).

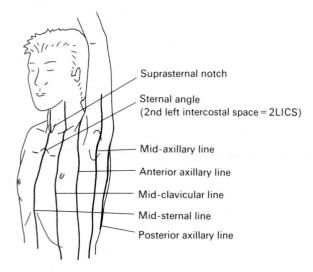

Suprasternal notch

Sternal angle
(2nd left intercostal space = 2LICS)

Mid-axillary line

Anterior axillary line

Mid-clavicular line

Mid-sternal line

Posterior axillary line

Fig. 8.   Landmarks of the precordium.

2 The 'v'-wave which is caused by venous filling and corresponds with ventricular systole. It coincides with the carotid pulse and with ventricular impulse felt at the apex beat. The 'v'-wave will be:

● Increased in tricuspid regurgitation.

3.5   Examination of the Precordium

Inspect for
  Abnormal pulsation
  The apex beat
Palpate
  The apex beat
    position
    character
  Other impulses, heaves
  Thrills

Describe in relation to the imaginary lines shown in Fig. 8
Percussion is not usually helpful

The apex beat

This is the outermost and lowest pulsation palpable and is normally in the 5th intercostal space (ICS) internal to the mid-clavicular line (MCL). It usually corresponds to the apex of the left ventricle and its character is determined by a combination of the contraction of the ventricle itself and the degree of rotation of the heart in systole. The apex beat may be difficult to locate in obese, muscular or emphysematous individuals. The patient may be asked to turn on his* left side to facilitate assessment of the character of the apex beat but its position will be altered.

Cardiac enlargement or mediastinal displacement may affect the **position** of the apex beat so it is important to determine that the trachea is central before interpreting the position of the apex beat.

The following may cause displacement of the apex beat:

- Congenital – skeletal abnormalities, dextrocardia
- Extrinsic – tension pneumothorax, pleural effusion
  pulmonary fibrosis, lung collapse
- Intrinsic – left ventricular hypertrophy or dilatation

Document the position with reference to intercostal spaces and clavicular or axillary lines.

The **Character** of the apex beat may be documented as follows:

- Heaving, diffuse – suggests left ventricular dilatation caused by aortic or mitral incompetence
- Forceful, localised – suggests concentric hypertrophy as in aortic stenosis, systemic hypertension
- Tapping – the palpable first heart sound of mitral stenosis

Other impulses

Pulsation:

- Under the left costal cartilages (parasternal heave) suggests right ventricular enlargement;
- In the 2nd and 3rd left intercostal spaces suggests pulmonary artery enlargement;
- In the 2nd right intercostal space suggests ascending aortic aneurysm.

A **double impulse** at the apex suggests left ventricular aneurysm. When palpable an exaggerated impulse is termed a 'heave'. A thrill is a palpable murmur and is always of pathological significance.

Percussion

The extent of cardiac dullness as determined by percussion gives a very poor guide to the size of the heart. However, a dull percussion note over the 2nd left intercostal space suggests pericardial effusion.

3.6   Auscultation of the Heart

Time all cardiac events by palpating the carotid pulse at the same time as listening to the heart. The first heart sound corresponds (almost exactly) with the carotid pulse and the onset of systole.

Listen in the following areas which classically (but not reliably) correspond with the maximum intensity of the valves.

'Mitral'	–	*at the cardiac apex*
'Tricuspid'	–	*to the right of the lower end of the sternum*
'Aortic'	–	*to the right of the sternum in the 2nd intercostal space*
'Pulmonary'	–	*to the left of the sternum in the 2nd intercostal space*

The first heart sound is usually most easily identified over the cardiac apex and this should be the first area to be auscultated. Then with the stethoscope proceed towards and then up the left sternal edge to the second left intercostal space and then across the sternum to the second right intercostal space and finally to the lower end of the sternum on the right. Follow the sound of any murmur in the direction of its transmission.

Identify and assess the first heart sound. Note whether it is:
normal, loud, soft, absent, split.

Identify and assess the second heart sound. Note whether it is:
normal, loud, soft, absent, split.

Listen carefully to the space between the first and second heart sounds (systole).

Is it quiet, or is there a murmur or other heart sound?

Listen carefully to the space between the second and first heart sounds (diastole).

Is it quiet, or is there a murmur or other heart sound?

If a murmur is present note

● *Timing* – *whether systolic, diastolic or throughout the cardiac cycle*

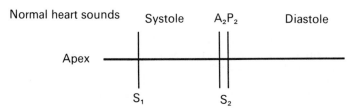

Fig. 9. Normal heart sounds.

- *Duration* – *whether at the beginning, middle, end or throughout either systole or diastole*
- *Character* – *described using words such as harsh, blowing, rumbling*
  - – *Same intensity throughout systole (pansystolic or holosystolic) or increasing and decreasing (ejection)*
- *Pitch* – *low or high*
- *Intensity* – *usually graded out of 4 or 6 with the higher number being louder.*
  - – *there may be an associated thrill.*
  - – *reduced when chest wall is thick or with emphysema*
- *Location* – *site of maximum intensity*
- *Extent and direction of transmission*
- *Influence of respiration and position*
- *Associated features*

If another heart sound is present note

- *Timing* – *whether systolic or diastolic and relation to valve sounds*
- *Character and pitch*

Document the heart sounds and added sounds (see Fig. 9).

First heart sound (S1)

This is caused by closure of the mitral and tricuspid valves. It is best heard medial to the cardiac apex at the lower sternal border.

The first sound is:

- Loud in mitral stenosis, tachycardia and hyperdynamic circulation
- Soft in bradycardia, left ventricular failure, mitral regurgitation
- Split in tricuspid stenosis, right bundle branch block (delay in tricuspid component).

Second heart sound (S2)

This is caused by closure of the aortic (A2) and pulmonary (P2) valves. Usually it is split with aortic closure occurring before pulmonary because of the pressure difference between the aorta and pulmonary arteries. The two components are best heard in the 2nd intercostal space to the left and right of the sternum respectively. The second heart sound will be:

- Loud A2 in systemic hypertension
- Soft A2 in aortic stenosis.
- Loud P2 in pulmonary hypertension
- Split S2 with splitting normally increased on inspiration because of delayed closure of pulmonary valve as blood is drawn into the right ventricle (RV).
  Wide splitting and no variation with respiration occurs in atrial septal defect (ASD).
  Reversed splitting (narrows on inspiration) is found in left bundle branch block because of delay in left ventricular (LV) contraction.

Third heart sound (S3)

This is a diastolic sound due to passive ventricular filling and occurring early in diastole (soon after S2). It may be heard in normal children and young adults particularly after exercise, but in other circumstances S3 suggests impaired left ventricular function.

Fourth heart sound (S4)

This is a late diastolic sound (heard just before S1) caused by rapid influx of blood into the ventricle during atrial contraction (therefore not heard in atrial fibrillation). It is rarely heard in health and suggests resistance to ventricular filling usually due to impaired left ventricular function.

The cadence caused by the addition of a third or fourth HS to the normal heart sounds is called a gallop rhythm (see Fig. 10).

An opening snap (OS) occurring soon after the second HS is heard in mitral stenosis.

Pericardial friction rub is a creaking sound heard in both systole and diastole and often modified by posture and respiration. It suggests pericarditis which may be due to:

- Viral pericarditis
- Myocardial infarction

Gallop rhythm

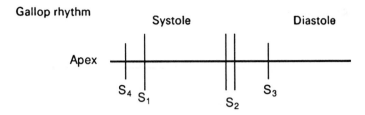

Fig. 10. Gallop rhythm.

- Connective tissue diseases
- Trauma
- Uraemia

There may be an associated pericardial effusion.

Systolic click may be heard in aortic and pulmonary stenosis and also (characteristically) in mitral valve prolapse.

Heart murmurs

You will already have some idea of the type of valve lesion to expect having noted abnormalities in the arterial and venous pulses and displacement of apex beat.

Commonly encountered **systolic murmurs** (with their characteristic features, see Fig 11) include:

- *Functional or physiological caused by increased flow through a normal heart*
  Never diastolic
  Short, soft, mid-systolic
  Localised usually to left sternal edge or apex
  Often diminished in intensity by sitting
  No associated cardiac symptoms or signs

- *Aortic stenosis*
  Initially mid-systolic but may extend throughout systole
  Harsh, high pitched (best heard with diaphragm), ejection
  Located at 2nd right intercostal space
  Radiates to both carotid arteries and sometimes to the apex
  Accentuated by leaning forwards in expiration.

Aortic stenosis

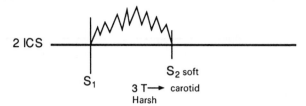

Mitral regurgitation

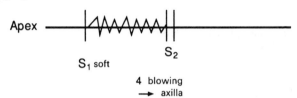

Mitral valve prolapse

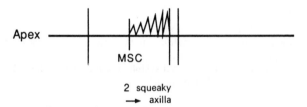

Fig. 11. Documentation of common heart murmurs.

- *Mitral regurgitation*
  Pan-systolic
  Blowing
  Located at the apex with radiation towards the axilla

- *Mitral valve prolapse*
  Mid-systolic click with variable degree of mitral regurgitation
  When regurgitation is mild the murmur is late systolic (occurring after the click) and tends to increase in intensity towards S2
  Mitral valve prolapse syndrome (Barlow's syndrome) tends to occur in thin individuals who are often anxious and have associated palpitation and non-ischaemic chest pain

Aortic regurgitation

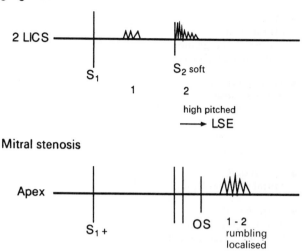

Fig. 11. (cont).

Commonly encountered **diastolic murmurs** (with their characteristic features) include:

- *Aortic regurgitation*
  Early diastolic starting immediately after S2
  Initially short but with valve incompetence more severe, may extend throughout diastole
  High pitched best heard at the left sternal edge with patient leaning forwards in expiration.

- *Mitral stenosis*
  One of the most difficult murmurs to hear
  Mid-diastolic with pre-systolic accentuation in sinus rhythm
  Low pitched, rumbling
  Localised to apex with no radiation
  Best heard with patient lying on his* left side preferably after exercise
  Associated with small pulse, opening snap, loud S1 and tapping apex beat.

The origin of some cardiac murmurs is as follows:

- *Pan-systolic*
  Mitral regurgitation
  Tricuspid regurgitation
  Ventriculoseptal defect

- *Ejection (systolic)*
  Aortic stenosis
  Pulmonary stenosis
  Atrioseptal defect (pulmonary flow)
  Hyperdynamic circulation
  Physiological

- *Late systolic*
  Mitral valve prolapse

- *Early diastolic*
  Aortic regurgitation
  Pulmonary regurgitation

- *Mid-diastolic*
  Mitral stenosis
  Tricuspid stenosis (very rare)
  Large atrioseptal defect

- *Continuous*
  Patent ductus arteriosus

3.7   Minimal statement of the cardiovascular system (CVS)

Pulse 80/min, regular
BP 120/80 right brachial, sitting
JVP not raised (JVP⁰)
No oedema (oedema ⁰)
Apex beat 5ICS, MCL
No evidence of right or left ventricular enlargement (RV + ⁰, LV + ⁰)
HS normal, no murmurs, no added sounds (or, as shown in Fig. 12)
Peripheral pulses present and equal (PP =)

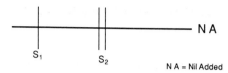

N A = Nil Added

Fig. 12. No added heart sounds.

Fig. 13. Documentation of common heart murmurs.

Documentation	Interpretation
Aortic stenosis 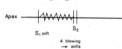	There is a grade 3 harsh ejection systolic murmur associated with a thrill heard loudest at the 2nd right intercostal space with radiation to the carotid arteries. The first heart sound is normal but the second is soft with loss of physiological splitting.
Mitral regurgitation 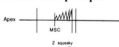	There is a grade 4 blowing pan-systolic murmur heard best at the cardiac apex with radiation to the axilla. The first and second heart sounds are soft.
Mitral valve prolapse 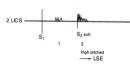	There is a late systolic murmur which increases in intensity and is squeaky in character heard best at the cardiac apex and with radiation to the axilla. There is also a mid-systolic click.
Aortic regurgitation 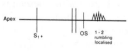	There is a grade 2 high-pitched immediate decrescendo diastolic murmur heard best at the 2nd left intercostal space with radiation along the left sternal border. There is also a short mid-systolic grade one murmur. The second heart sound is soft and single.
Mitral stenosis	There is a soft (grade 1 to 2) low-pitched rumbling mid-diastolic murmur localised to the cardiac apex with no radiation. The first heart sound is loud and there is an opening snap.

4   Examination of the respiratory system

4.1   General

The presence or absence of cyanosis and clubbing will already have been noted during the general examination.
   Note the following:

   Respiratory rate counted when the patient does not think that he* is being observed
   Respiratory rhythm
   Use of accessory muscles of respiration
   Conscious level

Respiratory rate

In an adult the respiratory rate is normally between 12–15/min and is best counted before the patient is approached or during another part of the physical examination (such as counting the pulse). The rate is increased in pneumonia, anxiety, acidosis and in the presence of pleuritic pain when respiration is rapid and shallow, being limited by the pain. Respiratory rate is decreased in narcotic overdose and hypoventilation due to cerebral or respiratory disease. Breathing through pursed lips is seen in chronic obstructive pulmonary disease and flaring of the alae nasi is a feature of pneumonia.

Respiratory rhythm

This varies considerably in both health and disease. Normally respiration is regular with occasional deep breaths that expand the lung bases. Sedation will abolish these breaths and predispose to the development of basal pneumonia (post-operatively for example).
   Cheyne-Stokes respiration has a very characteristic pattern in which successive breaths become deeper until a maximum is attained when there is a period of apnoea, and the cycle repeated. There are many causes but the patient is usually unconscious with serious cerebral or metabolic disorder.

Accessory muscles

The muscles of normal respiration are the diaphragm which descends on inspiration and causes outward abdominal movement, and the intercostals which cause chest expansion. In respiratory distress the neck muscles are recruited to lift the thorax and, not infrequently, the patient will be sitting forwards with arms folded on a table in front of him* to give additional purchase to the respiratory muscles.

Conscious level

Drowsiness leading to coma is seen in carbon dioxide retention from hypoventilation. Sweating, twitching and anxiety are features of hypoxia.

4.2   Inspection of the Chest

The front of the chest should be examined first (with the patient lying at 45°) and then the back (with the patient sitting upright). Note the following:

Shape of the chest
Symmetry and extent of the movements
Intercostal recession
Dilated veins
Operation scars

Chest shape (Fig. 14)

- **Kyphosis** is exaggerated antero-posterior curvature of the spine.
- **Scoliosis** is lateral curvature of the spine. This may be apparent only as an 'S' shape of the thoracic spine but as the condition progresses the vertebral bodies are rotated so that the ribs protrude backwards causing a 'hunch-back'.
- **Pectus excavatum** is depressed sternum.
- **Pectus carinatum** (pigeon chest) is protruberant sternum.
- **Barrel-shaped** chest is seen in the end stages of chronic obstructive pulmonary disease.

Chest movements

In the absence of spinal deformity, diminished movement on one side indicates disease on that side – increased movement is never pathological. If in doubt about the adequacy of chest movements, measure the chest circumference at nipple level with a tape measure on inspiration and expiration. The difference should normally be in excess of 5 cm.

Intercostal recession

A drawing-in of the intercostal spaces with inspiration indicates airway obstruction and non-compliant lung.

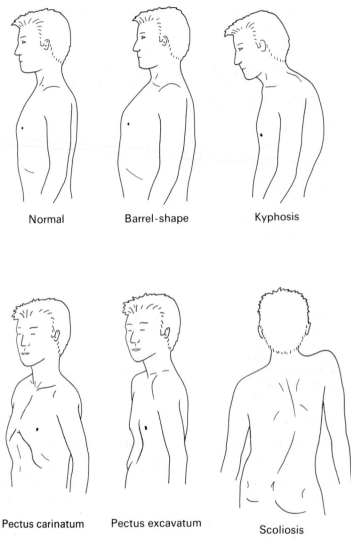

Normal   Barrel-shape   Kyphosis

Pectus carinatum   Pectus excavatum   Scoliosis

Fig. 14. Chest shape.

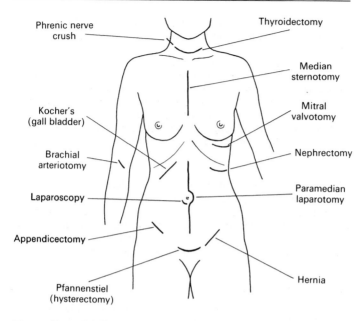

Fig. 15. Operation scars.

Operation scars (Fig. 15)

Operations were frequently performed before the mid-1950s as treatment for tuberculosis (before antibiotic therapy was introduced). A scar in the neck suggests phrenic nerve crush and there may be the scar and chest deformity of thoracoplasty. In addition there may be the scars of mitral valve surgery and the more modern mid-line sternal scar of coronary artery surgery or heart valve replacement.

4.3   Palpation of the chest

Check that the trachea is central using the tips of your second and third fingers to note the position of the trachea in the suprasternal notch in relation to the medial ends of the clavicles.
    Assess the movements of the chest by placing the palms of both hands on either side of the mid-line with fingers apart and thumbs together and feeling the symmetry of expansion as the

patient breathes in and out. A rough assessment of expansion may be made by observing how far the two thumbs separate on inspiration.

Check the position of the apex beat.

Compare the tactile vocal fremitus (TVF) on the two sides at two or three levels by placing the hand lightly on the chest, and asking the patient to repeat a resonant word (ninety-nine or one-one) and feeling transmission of the vibration.

If the complaint is of superficial chest pain, note any local rib tenderness (due to rib fracture, tumour or underlying pleurisy).

Trachea

The trachea may be pulled to one side by a collapsed lung or fibrosis (particularly affecting the upper lobes) and may be pushed to the opposite side by pleural effusion or pneumothorax. In addition the trachea may be displaced by tumours of the neck or upper mediastinum. Displacement of the apex beat when the heart size is normal suggests mediastinal displacement which may be accompanied by displacement of the trachea.

Tactile vocal fremitus

This is increased over consolidated lung and diminished when air, fluid or thickened pleura separates the lung from the chest wall, or when a major bronchus is occluded.

4.4   Percussion of the chest

Percuss the chest at several levels (four or five), comparing one side with the other including the clavicles (direct percussion of the clavicles with one finger should be gentle). Note the lower limits of pulmonary resonance on each side. This is much easier on the right side, where lung resonance gives way to liver dullness, than on the left where the lung resonance gives way to tympany of the stomach and large bowel. If there is concern that there may be lung which is dull to percussion at the right base it is useful to ask the patient to breathe in when the dullness due to the liver will disappear as it moves downwards with inspiration.

The percussion note is determined by the thickness of the chest wall, by the aeration of underlying lung and by any structures intervening between the lung and the chest wall.

Percussion note is:

- Resonant over normal lung
- Dull over solid lung (consolidation) or pleural thickening
- Stony dull over fluid (pleural effusion)
- Hyper-resonant over hyper-inflated lung (such as emphysema when cardiac and hepatic dullness will also be lost) or pneumothorax.

Auscultatory percussion involves gentle percussion over sternum with simultaneous auscultation of lung fields over the back of the chest; when increased this may indicate small areas of consolidation. A characteristic tympanitic resonance may be heard over pneumothorax when percussion is performed over the chest with two coins ('coin sound').

4.5   Auscultation of the chest

Breath sounds (BS)

> *Vesicular (normal)*
> *Bronchial*
> *Diminished*
> *Vocal resonance*
> *Whispering pectoriloquy*

Compare the breath sounds on the two sides of the chest at three or four levels using either the bell or the diaphragm.

Added Sounds

> *Crackles*
> *Wheeze*
> *Stridor*
> *Rub*

Breath sounds

The turbulent flow of air in the trachea and large airways generates 'white noise'. By the time the air has reached the 15th division of the bronchial tree the flow is laminar and no noise is generated. From this point distally the 'white noise' is modified by normal lung tissue which acts as a filter and attenuates the lower frequencies. These modified sounds heard with the stethoscope on the chest wall are the **normal or vesicular** breath sounds. They differ from the sounds heard over the trachea by being less harsh because the lower frequencies have been attenuated, and the inspiratory phase is continuous with the expiratory phase which is shorter.

When the 'white noise' is modified by abnormal (usually consolidated) lung the upper airway sounds are transmitted relatively unchanged and are heard over the chest wall as **bronchial breathing**. These sounds are harsh and there is a gap between inspiratory and expiratory phases which are equal in duration. An imitation of bronchial breathing may be obtained by placing the bell of the stethoscope over your temple and breathing with your mouth open. Bronchial breathing is heard over consolidated lung and also at the upper level of a pleural effusion.

The breath sounds are **diminished** when thickened pleura, air or fluid separates the lung from the chest wall, and in thick-set muscular or obese individuals. They are also diminished when the respiratory flow rate is considerably reduced as in severe asthma and occasionally when the relevant major bronchus is obstructed. Do not describe diminished breath sounds as 'diminished air entry' as this is not necessarily true. The intensity of the breath sounds heard at the chest wall may not accurately reflect airflow.

Speech will be modified by normal and consolidated lung in the same way as the white noise generated by breathing. Normal speech ('one-one-one' or 'ninety-nine') is muffled and indistinct when heard at the chest wall through normal lung tissue but is heard clearly through consolidated lung **(vocal resonance)**. A soft whisper is not normally heard at all at the chest wall but clearly audible when transmitted through consolidated lung **(whispering pectoriloquy)**. These two signs serve to confirm the presence of bronchial breathing and need not be sought routinely.

Added sounds

Crackles are non-musical explosive sounds caused by the rapid movement of air which occurs when an airway opens and there is equalisation of pressure. The distal airway opens with a 'pop'. In general, the coarser the crackle the larger is the obstructed airway, and the later in inspiration that the crackle occurs the more distal is the airway that is opening (the airways inside the thorax open with inspiration).

Conditions associated with airways closure include:

- Pulmonary oedema
- Pulmonary fibrosis
- Pneumonic consolidation (fine, late crackles)
- Bronchiectasis
- Chronic bronchitis (coarser, later crackles)

It is important to auscultate after asking the patient to cough as some crackles caused by physiological airway closure may disappear. In addition, remember that any patient who is unwell and not breathing deeply enough to expand and ventilate the lung bases will have basal crackles which may be unilateral if the patient tends to lie on one side.

Wheeze is the musical sound made by air passing through an airway that is narrowed and on the point of closure. The sound is caused by vibration of the wall of the airway, and the pitch will depend on the volume of tissue that is vibrating. In general the lower the pitch the larger is the airway. Wheeze usually occurs on expiration when the intrathoracic airways tend to close.

High-pitched polyphonic expiratory wheeze is characteristic of narrowing of multiple distal airways as in asthma. If the airways are so narrowed as to be occluded then there will be no airflow and therefore no wheeze.

Lower pitched monophonic wheeze (usually localised) suggests narrowing of a single larger airway, such as occurs with tumour, foreign body or inspissated mucus.

Stridor is a monophonic wheeze which is heard on inspiration and arises from a narrowed airway outside the thorax (usually trachea) that tends to close on inspiration.

Pleural rub is a sound likened to creaking leather which is thought to be generated by inflamed pleural surfaces rubbing against each other during respiration. The inflammation may be due to infection, autoimmune disease or pulmonary infarction.

4.6   Special tests

Sputum examination
Peak flow recording
Vitalography before and after inhaled bronchodilator
Flow-volume loop
Carbon monoxide transfer factor
Arterial blood gas measurements
Chest radiograph

Signs useful in differentiating between respiratory conditions (see Table 2).

Table 2. *Clinical signs of common chest disorders*

Disorder	Movement	Percussion note	Breath sounds	Added sounds	Other
Acute asthma	Symetrically reduced	Normal or hyper-resonant	Normal or reduced	Polyphonic wheeze + +	
Collapse	Reduced	Dull	Diminished	None	Trachea deviated towards lesion
Consolidation	Reduced	Dull	Bronchial	+/− Crackles	Whispering pectoriloquy Vocal resonance
Emphysema	Symetrically reduced	Hyper-resonant Absent cardiac and liver dullness	Normal or reduced	Occasional expiratory wheeze	Hyper-inflated chest
Pleural effusion	Reduced	Stony dull	Absent (Bronchial at upper limit of effusion)	None	Trachea deviated away from effusion
Pneumothorax	Reduced or absent	Hyper resonant Coin sign +	Diminished	None	Trachea deviated away from pneumo-thorax
Pulmonary fibrosis	Symetrically reduced	Normal	Normal	Fine late inspiratory crackles + +	

4.7   Minimal statement of the respiratory system examination (RS)

Respiratory rate 16/min, no distress
Chest shape normal
Trachea central
Movements =, expansion 6 cm
Percussion note resonant all areas†
Breath sounds vesicular, no added sounds†

† As a rule it is unlikely that there is significant lung disease present if percussion note and breath sounds are normal, so demonstration of the other clinical signs is not usually necessary.

---

5   Examination of the alimentary system (AS)

5.1   General

The presence or absence of anaemia, jaundice, spider naevi, palmar erythema, leuconychia, gynaecomastia, koilonychia, left supraclavicular lymph nodes, and the skin rashes associated with certain gastrointestinal conditions will already have been noted during the general examination.

In addition, look for asterixis by asking the patient to extend his* arms with hands cocked up and observe the brief downward 'flapping' motion of his* hands.

Asterixis

This is also called 'liver flap' but occurs not only with hepatocellular failure but also with renal and respiratory failure.

5.2   Inspection of the oropharynx

- *Lips*
  Angular stomatitis, cheilosis
  Herpes labialis

- *Gums*
  Spongy, hypertrophied

- *Oral mucosa (use a wooden spatula)*
  Pigmentation
  Ulceration

- *Teeth*
  Caries, false teeth (dentures)

- *Tongue*
  Dry, atrophic, furring, candida

- *Fauces, tonsils and palate.*

Lips, gums, oral mucosa

Soreness at the corners of the mouth (**angular stomatitis**) or cracked lips (**cheilosis**) suggests iron or vitamin deficiency (sometimes associated with malabsorption). The commonest cause however, is ill-fitting dentures.

Herpes labialis ('fever blister') is caused by *Herpes simplex* virus, type I and affects nearly half of the population (particularly women). The vesicular lesions form on the outer third of the upper or lower lip near the mucocutaneous junction and often recur at intervals of between 1 and 4 months. Recurrences may be precipitated by exposure to ultraviolet light, acute illness (such as pneumococcal pneumonia) and stress. Symptoms of burning or itching precede the appearance of vesicles by about 12 h, and the vesicles crust and heal without scarring in about a week.

Spongy, bleeding gums suggests poor dental hygiene but may indicate leukaemia or vitamin C deficiency. Hypertrophy of the gums (which does not occur in edentulous persons) may be a side-effect of prolonged phenytoin, cyclosporin or nifedipine therapy. If the hypertrophy is localised to one or more teeth it is likely to be due to periodontal infection (epulis).

Dark pigmentation inside the cheeks (buccal pigmentation) suggests hypoadrenalism (Addison's disease).

Aphthous ulceration may affect up to half of the population and is more common in women. The ulcers are shallow with a grey base, regular border and surrounded by a narrow margin of erythema. They may occur anywhere in the mouth and a history of recurrence is always obtainable. The lesions persist for up to 2 weeks and heal without scarring. Usually no systemic association is found but recurrent aphthous ulceration may indicate the presence of coeliac disease or inflammatory bowel disease.

Teeth

False teeth may be ill-fitting, or not worn at all, in which case there may be a risk of intestinal obstruction from inadequately chewed food. Dental caries and poor dental hygiene are important in the aetiology of infective endocarditis.

Tongue

Dryness of the tongue is a poor indicator of dehydration, the commonest cause being mouth breathing. Smooth, atrophic tongue (lack of papillae) suggests iron or vitamin B_{12} deficiency. Furring of the tongue is of little diagnostic value despite the popular lay view to the contrary. The 'fur' is due to accumulation of debris between the papillae and occurs in people without teeth (edentulous), heavy smokers and those who are too ill to move their tongue very actively in the mouth.

Infection with Candida (manifest as sore, white plaques which can be removed leaving a red, bleeding base) may occur after treatment with broad spectrum antibiotics, but may also be an important feature of Acquired Immune Deficiency Syndrome (AIDS) particularly if the Candida is extensive.

5.3   Inspection of the abdomen

Examine the abdomen in a good light with the patient lying as flat as is comfortable for him* with his arms by his* side and his legs uncrossed. Diagonal light is better than illumination from above. The patient's confidence must be gained if a satisfactory examination is to be made, and warm hands and gentle approach go a long way to securing this.

Expose the abdomen from xiphisternum to pubis, keeping the chest and legs covered with a sheet or blanket. Only expose the external genitalia when they are to be specifically examined. Inspect the abdomen from above and then with your eyes on a level with the abdomen (kneeling or sitting) noting any abnormality in the areas shown in Fig. 16.

Note:

- *Shape of abdomen and movements with respiration*

- *Distension*
  This may be in the flanks or in the central abdomen.
  Eversion of the umbilicus.

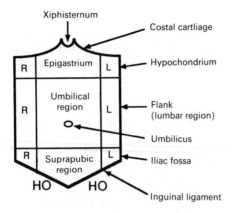

Fig. 16. Regions of the abdomen (HO, hernial orifice).

- *Operation scars (see Fig. 15, p. 101)*
  Many of the 'classical' abdominal operations now tend to be performed laparoscopically or with 'minimal invasion', thus leaving almost no scar.

- *Striae*

- *Visible peristalsis*

- *Distended veins and direction of flow.*
  Occlude a vein with a finger and with a second finger run along the vein away from the first finger so the blood is pushed out. When the first finger is released you can determine the direction of flow by seeing whether the vein fills.

- *Hernial orifices*

Shape

The abdomen may be slim (scaphoid) or covered by an apron of fat which makes examination very difficult. With advancing age and with osteoporosis the spine shortens and the costal margins approach the iliac crests, reducing the area to be examined.

The abdomen normally moves outwards with inspiration. Failure to do so suggests diaphragmatic paralysis or the muscular rigidity of peritonitis.

Distension

Abdominal distension may be:

- Localised due to an underlying mass, dilated loop of bowel, or, an enlarged abdominal organ
- Generalised due to free fluid in the peritoneal cavity (ascites) when distension will occur in dependent parts (fullness in the flanks), or generalised bowel dilatation when distension will tend to be central.
  Causes of generalised abdominal distension may be summarised as the 'five Fs' – fluid, foetus, faeces, fat, flatus.

The umbilicus will be everted when there is generalised abdominal distension or when there is an umbilical hernia.

Striae ('stretch marks') may be seen over the lower abdomen in women who have borne children (they are silver-grey colour). Rapid weight gain, corticosteroid treatment and Cushing's syndrome may cause red-purple ('active') striae.

Visible peristalsis may be seen normally in thin and elderly subjects. Otherwise, visible peristalsis indicates bowel obstruction. In the epigastrium peristalsis from left to right suggests gastric outlet obstruction, and from right to left transverse colon obstruction. Peristalsis seen over the central abdomen (ladder pattern) is due to small bowel obstruction.

Distended veins on the abdominal wall may occur normally in thin patients or during pregnancy. In portal hypertension there may be distended veins around the umbilicus (caput medusae) which represent anastomoses between the systemic and portal venous systems (also present in the oesophagus and stomach as varices and in the rectum as piles). Obstruction of the inferior vena cava causes distended veins over the abdomen due to blood being diverted from the saphenous vein to the axillary vein with the direction of flow being upwards.

5.4 Palpation of the abdomen

Ask if there is any abdominal pain and start palpation away from this area. Always look at the patient's face while palpating the abdomen because his* expression will tell you if this is causing discomfort.

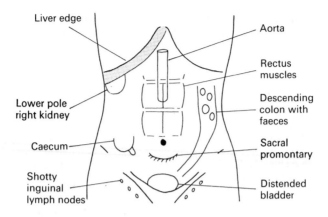

Fig. 17. Palpation of the abdomen – normal findings.

Palpate each quadrant superficially with a light touch to assess tenderness or guarding.
Then palpate more deeply to determine the presence of an abnormal mass or enlarged organ(s).
Characterise any mass by position, size, consistency, shape, and mobility (particularly in relation to respiration). Palpate liver, spleen, kidneys and bladder as part of the examination of these organs.
Test for gastric (succussion) splash. The abdomen is 'shaken' to and fro and the splash in the epigastrium is either felt or auscultated.
Palpate the hernial orifices; this is facilitated by asking the patient to cough but if a hernia is likely then the patient should be re-examined when standing.

Several normal structures may be palpated, particularly in slim subjects and those (often elderly) with lax abdominal musculature. These structures are shown in Fig. 17.

Localised or generalised **rigidity** (or 'guarding') is due to reflex contraction of the abdominal wall muscles to 'protect' an area of inflammation below and suggests local or generalised peritonitis. The rigidity may be palpated directly or be detected by holding your hand about 2 cm away from the abdominal skin surface and asking the patient to push his* abdomen out to touch your hand which he* will be unable to do. Alternatively ask the patient to pull in his* umbilicus.

If appendicitis is suspected, palpate **McBurney's point** (one third of the way along a line drawn from the right anterior superior iliac spine to the umbilicus). To determine whether mild degrees of tenderness or guarding indicate peritoneal inflammation, press your fingers gently into the tender area and then suddenly remove them. If removing the fingers in this way gives rise to pain (**rebound tenderness**), then this suggests peritoneal inflammation.

Succussion splash may be elicited over a normally full stomach, but if very obvious suggests pyloric outflow obstruction.

Indirect inguinal hernia passes through the internal inguinal ring along the inguinal canal, emerging through the external inguinal ring (above and medial to the pubic tubercle) and into the scrotum or labia majora.

Direct inguinal hernia passes through a defect in the posterior wall of the inguinal canal and, therefore, its path is forwards rather than diagonal. A finger inserted into the superficial inguinal ring passes directly backwards into the abdomen.

Femoral hernia emerges from the femoral canal which lies below and lateral to the pubic tubercle.

When a hernia is present, note whether coughing produces a palpable impulse (which excludes strangulation) and whether it is tender or reducible.

5.5   Percussion of the abdomen

Percussion is used to identify the presence of free or encysted fluid in the abdomen; to determine whether palpable tumours are superficial or deep; to help determine the size of the liver and spleen; to distinguish between retroperitoneal organs (such as kidney) which will be resonant because of the overlying bowel and liver which will be dull; and to identify an enlarged urinary bladder.

Shifting dullness is used to detect the presence of ascites. The fluid will collect in the dependent parts of the peritoneal cavity so if the patient is lying on his* back the fluid (and hence the dullness to percussion) will be in the flanks. If he* turns onto his* side then the fluid will again become dependent, leaving the upper flank resonant (i.e. the dullness has shifted). Percuss the area of dullness in the left flank and keep your finger over this *area. Ask the patient to roll onto his* right side so that your finger on his flank is uppermost and wait about 30 s (for the fluid to shift) and then percuss again without moving your finger. If the area is now resonant then you have demonstrated shifting dullness and the presence of free fluid in the peritoneum. This may be confirmed by asking the patient to lie again on his* back and confirm that the area is again dull to percussion.*

When the abdomen is distended with fluid, a fluid thrill may be demonstrated. This may be generated by tapping firmly on one flank and detected by feeling the thrill with the other hand placed on the opposite flank. The vibration from the tap is transmitted through the fluid but may also be transmitted through the fat of the abdominal wall. This can be prevented by asking an observer to press gently on the abdominal wall to stop transmission of the vibration through the fat.

The described technique of demonstrating shifting dullness will detect a minimum of about 2 litres. A smaller amount of ascitic fluid can be detected by demonstrating resonant percussion over the umbilicus with the patient lying on his* back and then putting him* in the knee–elbow position and percussing the abdomen from beneath. The fluid will collect around the umbilicus and give rise to an area of dullness (puddle sign) at this site. From a practical point of view a small amount of ascites is best demonstrated by ultrasound. The demonstration of a fluid thrill is not very helpful because the presence of ascites will usually be obvious.

5.6   Auscultation of the abdomen

Listen in the four quadrants of the abdomen and note the interval between intestinal sounds (borborygmi) and their pitch or the complete absence of sounds.
A bruit may be heard normally over the abdominal aorta in young, thin persons, but otherwise should suggest aortic aneurysm, or renal artery stenosis.

In **intestinal obstruction** the sounds are often more frequent, louder, high-pitched and tinkling. There may be a short period of quiet followed by loud sounds which coincide with severe colicky abdominal pain.

In **paralytic ileus** which may accompany generalised peritonitis, the sounds are absent and the abdomen is described as 'silent' although transmitted cardiac and respiratory sounds are often heard well.

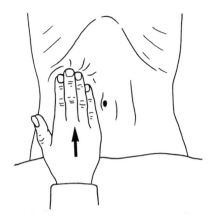

Fig. 18. Palpation of the liver.

5.7 Examination of the liver and gallbladder

Inspection

Note localised fullness in the right hypochondrium due to an enlargement of the liver. This may be more obvious if the abdomen is viewed horizontally rather than from above.
Spider naevi and fullness in the flanks (ascites) are associated with cirrhosis of the liver.
Distended veins may indicate portal hypertension.
Occasionally the distended gall bladder may be seen.

Palpation

The radial border of your right hand or your finger tips may be used to palpate the liver edge. Start in the right iliac fossa with the radial border of the hand parallel with the costal margin, or the finger tips pointing upwards (see Fig. 18).
Ask the patient to take deep breaths in and out and during the inspiration advance your hand towards the patient's chest at the same time as depressing it into the abdomen so as to feel the lower border of the liver as it descends.
If palpable, note the distance of the liver edge below the costal margin (in centimetres using the width of your finger as a guide)

in the mid-clavicular line or below the xiphisternum. Describe the consistency of the liver, the condition of its surface and edge and whether it is tender.

Percussion

This is useful to determine the size of the liver by defining the upper and lower liver margins (best carried out by percussing in the mid-axillary line to avoid breast tissue)and for confirming the position of the liver edge as determined by palpation. The upper border is identified by noting the change in percussion note from resonance over the lung to dullness over the upper border of the liver. The level of dullness will change with respiration and will normally be at about the fifth rib (nipple level) in the mid-clavicular line. The lower border is determined by percussion from the right iliac fossa and noting where the resonance of the bowel gives way to the dullness of the liver.

Auscultation

A friction rub may be audible over an hepatic infarct and frequently after percutaneous liver biopsy. Arterial bruits or a venous hum may be heard over a vascular tumour.
*The **scratch test** may be used to confirm the lower border of the liver. Place the diaphragm of the stethoscope over the liver above the costal margin and auscultate the sound made by scratching your finger over the abdominal wall. When the scratching finger overlies the liver the sound will change abruptly.*

The **liver** is not normally palpable although an extension to the right lobe (Riedel's lobe) may be felt. The liver may be of normal size but palpable below the costal margin because it is displaced by hyperinflated lung (e.g. emphysema).

Soft and tender hepatomegaly suggests hepatitis or heart failure. Firm and nodular enlargement suggests cirrhosis (in the early stages before the liver shrinks), metastases or primary hepatocellular carcinoma (hepatoma).

The following stigmata should be sought if **chronic liver disease** is suspected:

- Jaundice
- Clubbing
- Leuconychia
- Palmar erythema

- Spider naevi
- Scratch marks and bruising
- Gynaecomastia and atrophic testes

The **gallbladder** is not palpable unless enlarged and it may then be felt (often with difficulty) in the mid-clavicular line.

Corvoisier's Law states 'if in the presence of jaundice the gall bladder is palpable then the cause of the jaundice is unlikely to be a stone impacted in the common bile duct'. The reason is that gall stones will probably have caused previous cholecystitis leading to a small fibrotic gall bladder.

Cholecystitis may be detected by pressing the fingers gently into the right hypochondrium as the patient takes a deep breath in. A sudden catch of breath when the gallbladder touches your fingers indicates inflammation (**Murphy's sign**).

Hyperaesthesia over thoracic segments 9, 10 and 11 posteriorly on the right side (**Boas' sign**) is also a feature of gall bladder inflammation.

5.8   Examination of the spleen

Inspection

Fullness in the left hypochondrium may be observed when the spleen is very large.

Palpation

Start in the right iliac fossa and move your hand towards the left costal margin asking the patient to breathe deeply in and out, the hand should be pressing upwards during inspiration to catch the lower border of the spleen as it descends (Fig. 19). Frequently, it is only the tip of the spleen that is palpable and this emerges from the costal margin in the mid-axillary line (i.e. far more posterior than is usually appreciated).

If splenomegaly is anticipated but not detected in the supine position ask the patient to turn towards you (onto his* right side, Fig. 20) put his* left hand on your shoulder (or relaxed by his left side) and support the patient's back either with your left hand or with a pillow. Again, palpate the spleen which may be more easily felt in this position. It is important that palpation is gentle, because an enlarged spleen may be very fragile (particularly in infection such as glandular fever) and may rupture.

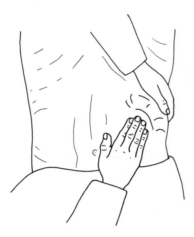

Fig. 19. Palpation of the spleen (patient supine).

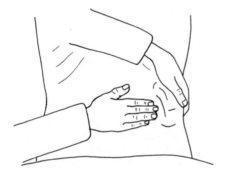

Fig. 20. Palpation of the spleen (patient lying on right side).

Percussion

The note will be dull over an enlarged spleen. If the percussion note over the lower ribs laterally on the left is resonant then it is unlikely that the spleen is enlarged.

Auscultation

This may demonstrate a friction rub over an area of splenic infarction usually in a greatly enlarged spleen.

In young subjects the spleen probably has to enlarge threefold before it is palpable but as the spleen shrinks in size with age this is not true of older subjects.

Causes of splenic enlargement include:

- *Huge spleen*
  Chronic myeloid leukaemia
  Myelofibrosis
  Kala-azar
  Lymphoma

- *Moderately enlarged spleen*
  Above list plus:
    Haemolytic anaemia
    Portal hypertension
    Storage diseases

- *Just palpable spleen*
  Above list plus:
    Infective endocarditis
    Infectious mononucleosis
    Typhoid

5.9 Examination of the kidneys

Inspection

This will demonstrate fullness in the flanks only in the case of very enlarged kidneys (such as polycystic kidneys).

Palpation

This is by ballottement bimanually. The flat of the left hand is placed in the loin posteriorly and the right (palpating) hand is placed anteriorly over the flank. The palpating hand is kept still and the kidney is pushed forwards by the posterior hand while the patient is asked to breathe in and out. An enlarged kidney is felt by the palpating hand.

Percussion

This will usually demonstrate resonance over an enlarged kidney (particularly the left) because bowel overlies the retroperitoneal organ.

The normal kidney is not usually palpable although the lower pole of the right kidney may be detected in thin subjects on inspiration. However, a kidney may be enlarged because of tumour, hydronephrosis (due to obstruction) or polycystic disease (bilateral).

Signs which help to distinguish between enlarged left kidney and enlarged spleen are:

- Left kidney is bimanually palpable, spleen is not
- Fingers can usually reach above upper pole of kidney, not so for the spleen
- Spleen has a notch on its medial border, kidney does not
- Spleen enlarges towards the right iliac fossa and the kidney towards the left iliac fossa
- Spleen tends to be dull to percussion and kidney resonant (unless very enlarged with displacement of overlying colon)

5.10   Examination of the urinary bladder

The enlarged bladder may be demonstrated by inspection (smooth swelling arising from the pelvis), palpation (tense, spherical, immobile swelling which you cannot get below) and percussion (stony dull).

The very full normal bladder may occasionally be demonstrated by palpation above the symphysis pubis. It will be tender and will stimulate the desire to void. Chronic distension of the bladder due to outflow obstruction (usually prostatic hypertrophy) is painless; the bladder may contain 4 litres of urine.

In women, the distended bladder has to be distinguished from an enlarged uterus (pregnancy or fibroids). The uterus is mobile laterally and may be felt bimanually on vaginal examination.

5.11   Digital examination of the rectum

This should be performed in all patients, but may be deferred, unless relevant, if the patient is very ill.

1. *Place the patient in a curled up position lying on the left side (left lateral position) and make sure that he* is covered with a sheet or blanket.*
2. *Examine the anus, noting whether there are any external hae-morrhoids, fissures or other abnormalities.*
3. *After inserting a gloved index finger (usually the right) covered with lubricating jelly, note the condition of the anal sphincter and*

the presence or absence of faeces in the rectum. In a male patient palpate the prostate (anteriorly) and describe its size and consistency and whether or not the median groove is palpable. A malignant prostate feels hard and woody and the median sulcus is often obliterated.

Do not confuse the normal cervix (felt anteriorly) with a tumour.

4. *If a tumour is felt, note its size, situation, consistency, shape and mobility.*
5. *Can pain be produced by pressure in any part of the rectum and if so in which direction?*
6. *Describe any other abnormality which can be felt.*
7. *Did examination cause bleeding?*

5.12 Examination of the external genitalia

Male

(chaperoned in the case of female students)

Note distribution of pubic hair (male escutcheon).
Note any obvious abnormalities of the penis.
Examine the scrotum and both testes (if absent seek along their line of descent).
Note testicular size and consistency.
Note any swellings.

Note small size of penis, penile discharge, hypospadias, phimosis (tight prepuce covering the glans), or paraphimosis (tight prepuce surrounding the base of the glans).

Normal adult testes are about 5 cm in length and are firm and not tender. The size of the testes may be assessed by comparing them with specially prepared oval wooden 'beads' usually strung together for convenience (orchidometer). Small, soft testes indicate cirrhosis or hypogonadism (e.g. Klinefelter syndrome). A testicular tumour may be impalpable and ultrasound is very useful.

Spermatocele is a retention cyst of the vasa efferentia lying above and behind the testis.

Hydrocele is due to accumulation of fluid within the tunica vaginalis which may almost surround the testis and which may be transilluminated when a lighted torch is pressed against it.

Varicocele is caused by varicosity of testicular veins, evident when the patient is standing.

Female

(only to be done when appropriate and when chaperoned in the case of male students)

> *Note distribution of pubic hair.*
> *Note obvious abnormalities of introitus.*
> *Note enlargement of clitoris.*
> *Vaginal examination should only be done in the presence of the House Officer and when appropriate.*

Extensive distribution of pubic hair over abdomen and a male escutcheon (hirsutism) is associated with alteration in oestrogen/androgen balance (e.g. polycystic ovary syndrome, adrenogenital syndrome). Enlargement of clitoris suggests androgen excess.

The stages of development of secondary sex characteristics may be documented using the standard ratings on a scale 1 to 5 as described in the Tanner-Whitehouse Growth and Development Record. The pubic hair development of both sexes is described from pre-adolescent (where the pubic hair is no different from that on the abdominal wall) to adult in quality, type and distribution. Genital development of boys is assessed by the change in appearance of the penis, scrotum and the size of the testes. There is no equivalent assessment of the genital development of girls but breast development is charted from pre-adolescent to maturity.

5.13   Minimal statement of the alimentary system examination

> Mouth, tongue, fauces and teeth – normal
> Abdomen – soft, no tenderness, guarding or rigidity
> Normal bowel sounds
> Liver, spleen, kidneys and bladder not palpable
> No abnormal masses felt
> Hernial orifices – normal
> Rectal examination (PR) – normal
> External genitalia normal

Or, see Fig. 21.

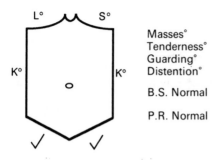

Masses°
Tenderness°
Guarding°
Distention°

B.S. Normal

P.R. Normal

Fig. 21. Examination of the alimentary system.

6 Examination of the nervous system

Obvious muscle weakness, involuntary movements and impairment of level of consciousness will already have been noted. The scheme given below is for a detailed general (rather than specialist) neurological examination. A 'screening' examination of the mental state, cranial nerves, limb power and reflexes will suffice when neurological disease is not anticipated (see Minimal statement of the nervous system, p. 161).

6.1 General

Note:
Appearance and position of patient
Conscious level
Facial appearance
Movements – voluntary, involuntary
Skull and neck – shape,
*   – listen for bruits*
*   – test for neck stiffness*
Kernig's sign
Spine – tenderness, shape (scoliosis, kyphosis), movements
Handedness (left or right)
Speech dysarthria
*   dysphasia*
*   dysphonia*

Appearance and position

A dishevelled and unkempt appearance suggests a chronic rather than acute neurological or psychiatric disorder.

A patient lying uncomfortably perhaps with a limb in a very awkward position suggests that he* may have focal weakness such as stroke.

For behaviour and emotional state assessment see Mental State at Interview. (See p. 25.)

Conscious level

The 'normal' state is one of unconsciousness and it is the reticular activating system in the brain stem (a physiological rather than anatomical entity) which leads to a state of alertness.

Depressed conscious level may be caused by:

- Brain stem dysfunction
- Focal abnormality of one cerebral hemisphere causing compression of the other hemisphere and of the brain stem
- Abnormality of function of both cerebral hemispheres, usually due to metabolic causes or drugs

Impaired consciousness varies from drowsiness to deep coma and is best described in terms of the degree and pattern of response to various stimuli, rather than using descriptions such as 'stupor' which may have variable interpretation.

The following may be used to describe increasing levels of impaired consciousness:

1. Fully alert and cooperative
2. Drowsy but becomes alert in response to verbal command
3. Unconscious but wakes and makes appropriate response to painful stimuli such as pressure over the supraorbital nerve in the supraorbital notch, forceful massage of the sternum, or pinching of the ear lobes.
4. Unconscious with incoordinated response to painful stimulus
5. Coordinated flexion response to pain (decorticate)
6. Coordinated extension response to pain (decerebrate)
7. No response to pain
8. Brain stem death

An objective and repeatable measure of the conscious level may be obtained from the Glasgow Coma Scale (see table) based on best response of eye-opening, speaking and movement to command as follows:

	Response	Score
Eye opening	Spontaneous	4
	To command	3
	To pain	2
	Nil	1
Verbal response	Orientated	5
	Confused conversation	4
	Inappropriate words	3
	Incomprehensible sounds	2
	Nil	1
Best motor response	Obeys commands	6
	Localises to pain	5
	Withdraws from pain	4
	Flexion to pain stimulus	3
	Extension response to pain	2
	No response to pain	1

The scores from each of the three sections are added together and this may be repeated at intervals to indicate a trend in the change in conscious level.

For the **diagnosis of brainstem death**:

- The patient must be unconscious and requiring ventilator support.
- Depression of conscious level by drugs must be excluded.
- Hypothermia, metabolic and endocrine causes for coma must be excluded.
- A firm diagnosis of irreparable brain damage should have been established.

Once these criteria have been fulfilled the following observations are made and tests performed and repeated after an interval:

1. The pupils are dilated and do not respond to light
2. There is no ocular response to application of ice-cold water to the tympanic membranes
3. Corneal reflexes are absent
4. There is no motor response in the cranial nerve distribution in response to pain
5. There is no response to tracheal and bronchial stimulation
6. There is no respiratory response to hypercapnoea ($pCO_2 > 6.7kPa$)

After the second set of tests the patient may legally be declared dead.

Facial appearance

Facial weakness may be due to:

- Upper motor neurone with sparing of frontalis, most usually due to stroke.
- Lower motor neurone such as Bell's palsy.

Myopathic facies (due for example to dystrophia myotonica) is characterised by bilateral ptosis, expressionless face with smooth forehead, drooping of the eyelids and jaw, often with drooling of saliva, and sunken cheeks.

Mask-like facies of Parkinson's syndrome where the face is expressionless and blinking is infrequent.

Movements

1. Voluntary

   Difficulty with fine movements such as undoing buttons in the absence of arthritis and muscle wasting suggests an upper motor neurone lesion.

   Note general mobility and whether one side of the body (or one arm or leg) is less mobile.

2. Involuntary

   - Tremor – repetitive, regular oscillation about a joint

     Fine suggests hyperthyroidism

     Coarse is seen in anxiety

     Rhythmical with frequency of about 5/s, particularly affecting the pronation/supination of the wrist is typical of Parkinson's disease/syndrome ('pill-rolling')
   - Athetosis – Slow, writhing movements
   - Chorea – Jerky, random, non repetitive movements
   - Tic (or habit spasm) – stereotyped and often complex jerking movements which may be voluntarily suppressed for a short time
   - Blepharospasm – repetitive, irregular muscle twitching particularly affecting the orbicularis oculi
   - Fasciculation – irregular, diffuse contraction of motor units within a muscle suggesting denervation.

Skull and neck

Note shape of skull. Auscultate with the bell of the stethoscope over parietal bones, exit foramina and orbits. Ask the patient to close both eyes and then place the stethoscope over one eyelid

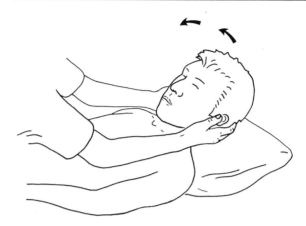

Fig. 22. Neck stiffness.

and ask the patient to open the other eye. This manoeuvre
reduces the movement of the eye under the closed eyelid and
prevents any bruit being obscured by the sound of muscle
contraction.
Auscultate with the diaphragm of the stethoscope over the neck
for bruits which may suggest carotid artery stenosis or arterio-
venous malformation for example.

*Check for **neck stiffness** due to spasm of the nuchal muscles*
(see Fig. 22). The examiner's hands are placed behind the
patient's head with the patient lying flat on his* back and an
attempt is gently made to flex the head (putting chin on chest).
Resistance to neck flexion (and discomfort) due to muscle spasm
occurs in the presence of meningeal irritation.

*Demonstrate **Kernig's sign**, which is the inability due to*
muscle spasm to extend the leg when the lower limb is flexed at
the hip (see Fig. 23).This procedure stretches the lumbar nerve
roots and is also a test of meningeal irritation.

***Meningeal irritation** is due to meningitis (either viral or*
bacterial), subarachnoid haemorrhage or 'meningism' which
occurs in the presence of severe febrile illness (pneumonia for
example), particularly in children. The patient will usually be lying
still in a quiet, darkened room because of increased sensitivity to

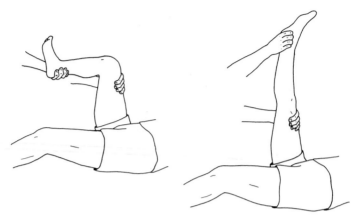

Fig. 23. Kernig's sign.

the light (**photophobia**) and in severe cases the neck and spine
are in a position of extension (**opisthotonus**).

Other causes of neck stiffness include painful cervical spine
lesions and severe pharyngitis but in these conditions movements
of the neck in all directions (not just flexion) will cause
discomfort and perhaps muscle spasm.

The features of meningeal irritation are:

- Headache
- Vomiting
- Photophobia
- Neck stiffness
- Positive Kernig's sign

The spine

Observe the undressed patient from behind.

Percuss the length of the spine (initially gently) noting any
tenderness.

Test movements of the cervical spine by asking the patient to
put his* chin on his* chest (flexion), look upwards (extension),
put ear on right then left shoulder (lateral bending) and finally,
twist head round to look over left and then right shoulder
(rotation). Care is needed when testing extension in the elderly as
such patients may become dizzy.

Test movements of the dorsal spine with the patient seated (to anchor the pelvis) and ask the patient to twist head and shoulders as far to the left and then right as possible.
Flexion of the lumbar spine is assessed with the patient standing and asking him* to touch his* toes with straight knees.
Test for tenderness of the sacroiliac joints by pressing firmly over the mid-sacrum with the patient lying prone.

Kyphosis (Fig. 14) is a flexion deformity, usually in the thoracic region. It may take the form of a smooth curve (osteoporosis, ankylosing spondylitis) or a sharp angle due to destruction of the vertebrae at one site (tuberculosis, metastases).

Scoliosis (Fig. 14) is a combined lateral and rotational deformity of the spine which if severe causes a 'hump back' with severe cosmetic and respiratory problems. Common causes in the past have included poliomyelitis and congenital abnormalities, but idiopathic scoliosis is now the most usual cause.

Reduced flexion of the spine (often associated with sacroiliac tenderness) is a feature of seronegative arthritis, particularly ankylosing spondylitis.

Speech

You will have listened to the content of speech while taking the history and noted neologisms (invented words) and circumlocution (roundabout explanation of a forgotten word) which suggest expressive dysphasia and difficulty with pronunciation (suggesting dysarthria). In addition, confabulation, delusions and hallucinations should become apparent.

Test for dysarthria by listening carefully to speech during the interview and asking the patient to repeat phrases and words such as
Baby hippopotamus
British constitution
Artillery

Dysarthria is a defect of articulation due to weakness or incoordination of the bulbar muscles or abnormalities of the tongue or lips, with preservation of language content. The following types are recognised:

- Stammer — a developmental abnormality of unknown cause.
- 'Baby speech' — which is usually loud and suggests profound deafness occurring before speech was fully developed.

- Scanning dysarthria — due to cerebellar dysfunction. The words are broken into separate syllables – for example artillery becomes ar-till-er-y
- Spastic dysarthria — due to pseudobulbar palsy. The consonants are slurred and the patient is often accused of being drunk.
  'British constitution' becomes 'Brish consh tushion'.
- Parkinsonian speech — is slow and lacks variation in pitch (monotonous).

Dysphasia is impairment in understanding or expressing language. In testing speech function, distinction must be made between dysphasia, dysarthria, confusion, clouding of consciousness (and occasionally a marked regional accent – dysprosody).

- *Expressive dysphasia is the inability to express by the spoken (or written) word. It may be apparent in conversation which may be limited to just 'yes' or 'no'. Test formally by asking the patient to explain the meaning of a simple proverb.*

Expressive dysphasia is due to a lesion of Broca's area in the tempero-parietal precentral gyrus (or a subcortical lesion cutting off Broca's area) and is sometimes called Broca's or motor dysphasia.

- *Receptive dysphasia is a failure to understand the spoken word or a command. Ask the patient to perform tasks of increasing complexity ensuring first of all that they are physically able to do so. Initially the command may be 'raise your left (non-paralysed!) hand' followed by increasingly more complicated commands such as 'touch your left ear with your left index finger'.*

Receptive dysphasia is due to a lesion of the posterior parietal angular gyrus and is sometimes called Wernicke's or sensory dysphasia. Speech is often fluent (because Broca's area is intact, but may be unintelligible because of the use of non-existent words (neologisms) and poor sentence construction (jargon aphasia).

- Global aphasia is the term used to describe the combination of receptive and expressive dysphasia as occurs with extensive cortical damage due to stroke.
- Nominal dysphasia is the inability to name objects (such as parts of a watch) and suggests a lesion of the temporal lobe.

Dysphonia is an abnormality of producing sound from the larynx and may occur with vocal cord palsy or laryngitis.

Test for impaired calculation. Ask the patient serially to subtract 7 from 100 and to continue until reaching 2.

Impairment in calculation (**dyscalculia**) suggests a parietal lesion often located in the non-dominant angular gyrus.

Dyslexia is a condition where the patient cannot recognise words, letters or colours. The lesion is in the dominant medial occipito-temporal (lingual) gyrus.

Dysgraphia is impairment of communication in the medium of writing rather than speech.

Test by asking the patient to write his* name and the answer to a question that you have asked him*, or ask him to write a sentence of his* choice, having told you what it should be.

6.2 Assessment of higher cerebral function

Formal assessment of higher cerebral function is usually unnecessary if an articulate history and a cooperative examination can be given by the patient. If conscious level is impaired, further tests of higher cerebral function are usually irrelevant.

If conscious level is normal test:
1 Orientation in time and place
   Ask the approximate current date. If the reply is completely incorrect then ask which month or season it is and the year.
   Ask the approximate time of day (without the patient looking at a clock or watch), with the response being either a time or an indication that it is morning or evening.
   Ask the patient to identify his* present location, the name of the hospital for example, or if he* is aware that he* is in a hospital.
2 Attentiveness
   Assess by digit span test. Normally six or seven figures can be remembered and immediately repeated.
3 Memory
   ● *Short-term memory is tested (assuming attention span is normal) by asking the patient to repeat a series of five, six or seven numbers in correct order, the normal digit span being six or seven figures.*
   Asking what the patient had for breakfast (and similar questions) may be useful in assessing short-term memory as long as it is possible to confirm that the answers are correct. Beware of confabulation, when the patient will give very plausible but totally fallacious answers.

- *Verbal memory is tested by recall of a name and address, by appreciation of recent current events, or being able to precis a short story. Repetition of the Babcock sentence ('The one thing a nation needs in order to be rich and great is a large, secure supply of wood') is the classical test as most subjects can repeat this after one or two hearings.*
- *Visual memory involves recognition of photographs of well-known personalities.*
- *Long-term memory is usually well preserved and can be tested by asking about past events. Elderly patients will often enjoy reminiscing and should be encouraged to do so.*
- *Reason and problem-solving may be subtly impaired in the absence of other derangement but may be difficult to demonstrate, as bedside tests are insensitive and the patient's attempts are influenced by IQ. Test by asking the patient to repeat four digits in reverse order or by asking how many 6p oranges can be bought for 40p.*

Patients with diffuse cerebral lesions, drug intoxication and certain metabolic disorders may be disorientated in time and place but still be alert.

Short-term and verbal memory loss may be due to a lesion of the temporal lobe or hippocampal region. **Korsakoff's psychosis** is a syndrome characterised by gross loss of recent memory with gaps in memory being filled by confabulation. The syndrome is usually associated with chronic alcoholism but may occur as a complication of other toxic and degenerative cerebral conditions.

Visual memory loss suggests a lesion of the right temporal lobe. Abnormality of reasoning suggests widespread cortical disease or frontal lobe dysfunction.

Dementia is the term applied to diffuse deterioration in mental function which is often first manifest as deterioration in thought and reasoning, and reduction in short-term memory. There are several causes but the commonest is Alzheimer's disease.

Cognitive skills are learned mental activities which at their most basic are the ability to speak, understand speech, read, write and perceive objects. These skills are related to the left hemisphere in 99% of right-handed subjects and 60–70% of left-handed subjects and are functions of the parietal and temporal regions. Assessment of these skills may have considerable localising value but of course the educational background of the subject must be taken into account when these functions are examined. The importance of establishing cerebral hemisphere dominance is obvious and thus 'handedness' should always be noted.

The **mental test score** using the Abbreviated Mental Test (AMT) (see table) is a rapid, objective and reproducible way of assessing cognitive function. Give one mark for each of the following (maximum score is ten):

Age
Time (to nearest hour)
Address for recall at the end of the test
The present year
Date of birth (day, month and year)
Name of place/hospital/institution
Recognition of two persons
Dates of First World War
Name of present monarch
Count backwards from 20 to 1

A score of 7 or less suggests significant impairment.

4 Examination of cortical motor function

Apraxia is a disturbance in the ability to perform a purposeful act when comprehension and motor and sensory function is intact and in the absence of ataxia. Any voluntary movement may be affected, the commonest being apraxia of the lips and tongue which frequently occurs in association with right hemiplegia from stroke. The patient may spontaneously lick his lips but will be unable to do so to command. Apraxia for dressing is often a problem after a non-dominant stroke.

***Constructional apraxia** is the inability to orientate in space. Ask the patient to copy a five-pointed star or join numbered dots in sequence (trail test). The advantage of the latter is that it may be timed, thus giving an objective measurement which may be compared on different occasions.*

Impairment suggests posterior parietal lesion or metabolic derangement such as hepatic encephalopathy.

***Grasp reflex** is elicited by firmly stroking the radial palmar surface of the patient's hand, moving distally between the thumb and forefinger. A positive (abnormal) response is that the examiner's hand is grasped, and this grip is maintained even if the patient is distracted.*

A positive grasp response is associated with diffuse cortical damage and particularly with disease of the contralateral frontal lobe.

6.3   Examination of the cranial nerves

I Olfactory nerve

Informal test – smell flowers or identify other smells on the ward. The sense of taste will often be lost if there is impairment of the sense of smell.
Formal test – smelling bottles (of four to six different types) or microencapsulated odorants mounted on a card and presented as a 'scratch and sniff' booklet.

The sense of smell is usually only tested formally when a frontal tumour (typically meningioma of the olfactory groove) is suspected or after a head injury. However, other causes of loss of smell (**anosmia**) include intranasal neoplasms and Kallman's syndrome (anosmia and hypogonadotrophic hypogonadism). It is the appreciation of smell by each nostril and not identification of smell that is important. Avoid using very pungent smells as these may be appreciated by the pain fibres of the trigeminal nerve. The commonest cause of impairment of smell is inflammation of the nasal mucosa due to upper respiratory tract viral infection.

II Optic nerve

1 Visual acuity
Allow patient to wear glasses if worn.
Rough test: reading (use newspaper or book)
Formal test: Jaegar card (near vision)
*   Snellen chart (distant vision)*
If acuity is severely impaired determine the degree by noting the patient's ability to count fingers, observe hand movements, and to perceive or not perceive light.

Refractive errors of the lens are the commonest cause of visual impairment and these may be corrected by asking the patient to repeat the test looking through a pin hole.

2 Colour vision
Rough test: equal appreciation of coloured object (red) by each eye
Formal test: Ischihara chart

Colour vision tends to be impaired early in the course of optic neuritis.

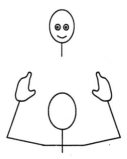

Fig. 24. Fields of vision: simultaneous movements in right and left fields.

3 Fields of vision

An approximate test of peripheral fields is by **confrontation** *comparing the field of vision of the examiner with that of the patient:*
Examiner and patient sit approximately 1 m apart facing each other.

The patient and the examiner keep looking at each other's nose and the examiner starts with arms outstretched and moves a finger (placed equidistant between himself* and the patient), starting at the periphery of his* field of vision and moving slowly towards the centre and asking the patient to indicate when he* can detect movement. This is repeated in the four peripheral quadrants.

Simultaneous movement of the fingers in the right and left fields will detect visual inattention in which the patient is able to detect movement on either the right or the left side but ignores one side when a stimulus is presented simultaneously (see Fig. 24).

Then the patient and the examiner each covers one opposing eye and stares into the opposite open eye of the other person (that is examiner's right eye and patient's left eye to start) and the procedure is repeated to exclude a monocular peripheral field defect (see Fig. 25). The test is repeated with the opposite eye.

The blind spot can also be plotted with the examiner comparing the size of his* blind spot with that of the patient.

Formal and more accurate testing of peripheral and central fields using a perimeter (e.g. Goldman) is performed in the eye

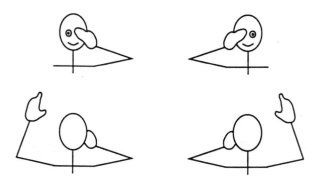

Fig. 25. Fields of vision: test for monocular defect.

clinic. The patient is presented with different sized targets in different parts of the visual field and a map of the fields of vision can be plotted.

Defects in the visual fields are of considerable localising value but it is very important to know the anatomy of the optic pathways.
Scotoma is a specific defect in the visual field due to damage to the nerve fibres of the macula. Optic neuritis is a common cause.
Bitemporal hemianopia occurs when the upward pressure of a pituitary tumour interferes with the blood supply of the optic chiasm.
Visual inattention is due to a dominant hemisphere parietal lesion.

4 Optic fundus using ophthalmoscope (Fig. 26)
The room should be darkened to enlarge the pupil and the patient's right eye should be examined with the ophthalmoscope applied to the examiner's right eye, and likewise the patient's left eye with the examiner's left eye. The ophthalmoscope should initially be set on a +20 dioptre lens and held 1 m from the pupil to assess the red reflex. Then advanced close to the patient's pupil with appropriate lens adjustment. It is sometimes helpful to view the optic fundus through the patient's spectacle lenses, particularly if they are strong lenses.
*   Identify the optic disc and then work peripherally along the vessels that radiate from the disc. Then identify the macula and visualise the remainder of the retina.*
Note:
Opacities in the cornea, anterior chamber, lens and vitreous humour.

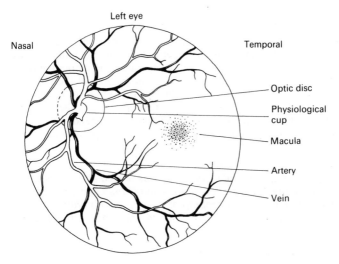

Fig. 26. The optic fundus.

Size, colour and contour of the optic disc and macula.
Distribution and size of retinal arteries and veins.
Presence of exudates, haemorrhages and pigment.

Black marks in the red reflex suggest lens opacities and cataract.

Papilloedema is a very important clinical sign. Initially the veins surrounding the optic disc become engorged and the disc (the optic nerve head) becomes pinker. The disc margins start to become blurred (the nasal edge of the disc is normally more indistinct than the temporal edge) and finally the whole disc becomes suffused and elevated.

Causes of papilloedema include:

- Raised intracranial pressure due to space occupying lesions (SOL), cerebral oedema or blocked circulation of cerebrospinal fluid.
- Malignant hypertension
- Metabolic disorders such as carbon dioxide retention
- Increased pressure within the orbit
- Disorders of circulation including retinal vein thrombosis.

Optic atrophy presents as a very pale optic disc and may follow papilloedema (secondary optic atrophy) or any toxic insult, demyelination from multiple sclerosis or retinal artery occlusion (primary optic atrophy).

III, IV, VI External ocular muscles (EOM)

Of these nerves, VI supplies lateral rectus muscle, IV the superior oblique and III supplies all the other muscles. In addition, the third nerve supplies the levator palpebrae superioris and carries parasympathetic fibres to the muscles of accommodation and the sphincter pupillae (constrictor). The afferent limb of the light reflex is conveyed in the optic nerve (II). Sympathetic dilator fibres to the sphincter pupillae arise in the cervical sympathetic chain and are conveyed to the eye with the internal carotid artery and thence the ophthalmic division of V.

*1 Examine eyelids for **ptosis***

When the eyes are fully open the upper eyelid should cover only the upper third of the cornea and should certainly not extend to the pupil. Drooping of the upper lid is often associated with overactivity of the frontalis in an attempt to lift the eyelid.

Unilateral ptosis may be due to

(i) A third nerve palsy. In addition to the ptosis there will be abnormal eye movements and dilated pupil.
(ii) **Horner's syndrome**. This is caused by a lesion of the sympathetic nerve supply to the eye and may occur anywhere along the pathway from the hypothalamus to the spinal root of T1 and up through the neck into the orbit.

The features of the syndrome in addition to the variable degree of ptosis are:

- constricted pupil which reacts normally
- impaired sweating of upper face
- enophthalmos (sunken eye) which is difficult to demonstrate clinically.

Bilateral ptosis is due to myopathy (such as dystrophia myotonica) but may be congenital (when it is often familial).

*2 Examine **pupils** for*
- *size and shape,*
- *reaction to light (direct and consensual) and*
- *reaction to accommodation/convergence*

First establish whether drops have been put into the patient's eyes. These may be therapeutic (for glaucoma causing pupil constriction) or diagnostic to cause pupil dilatation to aid fundoscopy.

To elicit the light reflex the patient should be in a dimly lit room and asked to look at a distant object (to eliminate the effect of accommodation). A bright light is brought in from the side to shine on the pupil and the constrictor effect on that eye (direct) and the other eye (consensual) is observed.

When the gaze is directed from a distant to a near object the pupil normally constricts. If both eyes are tested together (as is usual) the reaction is termed convergence and accommodation is used if each eye is tested separately.

Ask the patient to fix his* gaze on a distant object and then to look at your finger which is slowly brought to within about 5 cm of his* nose.

If the pupils are unequal in size it is important to establish which is the abnormal side by looking for ptosis or other abnormality. Many people have one pupil larger than the other and may have noticed this.

An irregularly shaped small pupil that reacts to accommodation but not to light (**Argyll-Robertson pupil**) suggests neurosyphilis (which is now very uncommon) or diabetes.

A moderately dilated pupil which fails to react to light and reacts slowly to accommodation may be associated with sluggish tendon reflexes and occurs particularly in women (**Holmes-Adie syndrome**).

Pinpoint pupils may occur with pontine haemorrhage in which case the patient is deeply unconscious with a spastic tetraparesis. Opiate use (or abuse) will cause pinpoint pupils and if there is coma the tendon reflexes will be depressed.

*3 Examine **eye movements** (Fig. 27) by first looking for a squint (**strabismus**) on forward gaze. The patient is asked to look at your finger held about 30 cm from his* nose. The visual axes should be parallel and, if not, then either convergent or divergent (according to the angle made by the ocular axes) squint is present.*

Then, ask the patient to follow your finger with his* gaze while you move it (always within his* field of vision) up and down, and to the right and left. It is usually necessary to fix the patient's head by gently holding his* forehead or chin with your other hand, and when observing downward gaze it helps to lift the upper eyelids.

Observe for conjugate eye movements and then the movements of each eye individually, with the other covered.

*While assessing eye movements look also for **nystagmus** which is a disturbance of ocular posture characterised by*

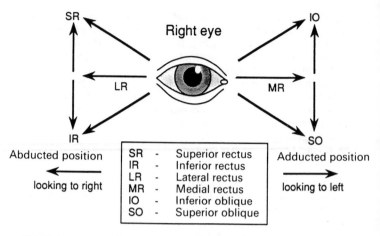

Fig. 27. Eye movements.

involuntary rhythmical oscillation of the eyes. The movements can be horizontal, vertical or rotary and may occur when the eyes are in a position of rest or only when looking in one direction. The quick phase is taken to indicate the direction of the nystagmus.

It is important not to extend the gaze outside the limits of binocular vision because nystagmus of no pathological significance may be produced.

Abnormalities of eye movements (**ophthalmoplegia**) may be due to:

- Conjugate ophthalmoplegia – often due to extensive (usually vascular) lesion of the cerebral hemisphere. The patient is usually unconscious and the head and eyes are turned to the side of the lesion.
- Internuclear ophthalmoplegia – usually producing dysconjugate lateral gaze (on attempted lateral gaze the contralateral medial rectus fails to contract even though it will respond normally on convergence) and characteristic of multiple sclerosis.
- Lesion(s) of one or more of the III, IV or VI cranial nerves (see diagram).

    For example:

    III paresis: eye points down and outwards (because of overaction of LR + SO)

    IV paresis: eye cannot look down and in

    VI paresis: eye cannot look laterally

- Abnormality of the ocular muscles themselves, for example in autoimmune thyroid disease.
- Concomitant squint which is one that is equal for all positions of the eyes and if the fixing eye is covered the movements of the squinting eye are full. There is no complaint of diplopia and the squint has usually been present since childhood.

Important **causes of nystagmus** are:

- Retinal disorders, usually impairment of macular vision of long standing. The nystagmus is usually horizontal and pendular with oscillations being equal in each direction and usually present on central fixation.
- Labyrinthine lesions, the nystagmus is usually rotary and may be due to acute lesions of the inner ear. Positional nystagmus is described later (VIII vestibular).
- Lesions of the brain stem and cerebellum (central), the nystagmus is most marked during conjugate eye deviation to the side of a unilateral cerebellar lesion and vertical nystagmus suggests a central brain stem lesion.
- Congenital and familial nystagmus which is often associated with albinism.

V Trigeminal nerve

Supplies sensation to the face (in three divisions) and cornea and motor fibres to the jaw.

1. *Test sensation of the face to light touch, pin-prick and temperature in the three divisions.*
2. *Test the corneal reflex – hold the lower lid down and ask the patient to look upwards and to the side. A wisp of cotton wool twisted to a point is brought up from below (so that the patient does not see it) and the lower, outer part of the cornea is gently stroked. Both eyes should shut simultaneously if the reflex is normal. If the reflex is difficult to demonstrate ask the patient if he* feels the stimulus to the cornea.*

    Ensure that the patient is not wearing contact lenses at the time of the test. The cornea of persons who wear hard contact lenses may be less sensitive.
3. *Examine the muscles of mastication*

    Look at the bulk of masseter and temporal muscles when the jaw is clenched. Ask the patient to close his* jaw while you exert downward pressure on the chin.

Assess the integrity of pterygoids by asking the patient to open his* jaw slowly against the resistance of a hand placed below the chin. If the right pterygoid is weak the jaw will open towards the right side.
4. The jaw jerk is elicited by asking the patient to open his* mouth slightly and relax his* jaw and then gently tapping your finger placed horizontally across his* chin with a patella hammer. A positive response is elevation of the jaw.

A pathologically exaggerated jaw jerk indicates an upper motor neurone lesion above the level of the pons. If the jaw jerk is normal but the tendon reflexes of the limbs are brisk, then the lesion lies below the foramen magnum.

Facial pain and abnormalities of facial sensation are common and noting that the corneal reflex is preserved is very important in assessing these symptoms. A reduced reflex suggests the possibility of a tumour (or other lesion) at the cerebro-pontine angle (acoustic neuroma for example).

VII Facial nerve

Supplies the frontalis muscle, the muscles of facial expression and platysma. There is no contribution to the upper eyelid so ptosis is not a feature.

Observe the face for asymmetry. When there is facial paralysis the affected side tends to droop and be pulled towards the stronger side. The creases of the forehead and the face (particularly nasolabial fold) will be smoothed out.
Assess the motor function of the upper face by asking the patient to

Screw up his* eyes
Raise his* eyebrows in surprise
Lower his* eyebrows in a frown

and the lower face by asking him* to

Show his* teeth in a smile
Whistle
Blow out his* cheeks against resistance

The upper part of the face is bilaterally represented in the cerebral cortex because reflex eye closure needs to be synchronised. Hence, unilateral weakness of the lower part of the face suggests upper motor neurone (UMN) lesion, whereas weakness of both upper and lower face (that is all muscles innervated by the seventh nerve) is due to a lower motor neurone (LMN).

Movements of the face with emotion tend to be spared in upper motor neurone lesions. Many patients have a degree of facial asymmetry, so it is important to ask the patient or a relative if there has been any change.

One of the most common acute neurological disorders is **Bell's Palsy** which consists of complete VII nerve palsy of LMN type which usually spontaneously recovers. The cause is unknown. Note **Bell's sign** – when asked to close his* eyes there is elevation of the eye on the paralysed side. A positive response involves the cornea being protected by the upper eyelid and this is important during sleep when the eyes are closed and the cornea may otherwise be exposed.

VIII Auditory nerve

Confirm that the patient can hear the sound of fingers rubbed together close to the ear or the ticking of a watch or whispered words.

*If hearing is impaired, compare air and bone conduction with a tuning fork (**Rinne's test**). Place a vibrating tuning fork (C = 256 or 512) over the mastoid process and then in front of the auditory meatus, asking the patient to say which he* hears better. Alternatively, the tuning fork is applied to the mastoid process until it is no longer audible (to the patient) when it should then still be audible at the external meatus.*

*In **Weber's test** the vibrating tuning fork is applied to the patient's forehead in the mid-line and he is asked if the sound is heard in the mid-line or localised to one ear.*

These tests must be combined with examination of external auditory meatus and drum with an auroscope.

Air conduction (AC) is normally better than bone conduction (BC) (noted as AC > BC) but will be impaired if there is conductive deafness due to obstruction of the external auditory meatus (wax) or middle ear disease. Normally sound is heard equally in each ear but if the sound is heard better in one ear it suggests either conductive defect in that ear or sensory nerve impairment in the other.

VIII Vestibular nerve

The vestibular nerve serves the vestibular apparatus (semi-circular canals and otolith organs) and has connections with the cerebellum. Abnormalities of the nerve may be associated with nystagmus, vertigo and ataxia.

- *Observe gait – patients with unilateral vestibular dysfunction tend to fall to the affected side (as they do with cerebellar dysfunction).*
- *Look for nystagmus – particularly with change of head position (positional nystagmus). The patient first sits and then is quickly lowered with his* head either to the right or left so that it rests below the horizontal over the edge of the couch. Acute vertigo with nystagmus occurs when the affected vestibular apparatus is in the underneath position.*

IX Glossopharyngeal nerve

The ninth nerve supplies sensation to the palate.

Test by touching the palate gently with an orange stick and comparing sensation on either side.

X Vagus nerve

The vagus is the motor nerve supplying the palate and vocal cords.
   Weakness of the palate may cause nasal regurgitation of fluid, nasal speech, hoarse voice and 'bovine' cough.

Observe the uvula and palate when the patient says 'aah'. The paralysed side will be pulled over towards the intact side.
   Ask the patient to cough.
   The movements of the vocal cords may need to be examined by direct or indirect laryngoscopy and this is best done by referral to the ENT clinic.

The **gag reflex** occurs when the palate or pharyngeal wall is stimulated which results in retching. The afferent arc is the IX nerve and the palatal movement and retching is mediated by the X nerve. It is an important protective reflex but is too inaccurate to be used for clinical diagnosis of specific cranial nerve lesions.

XI Spinal accessory nerve

This nerve is motor to the sternomastoid and trapezius muscles.

- *Observe wasting of sternomastoid and upper trapezius.*
- *Test the strength of trapezius by asking the patient to shrug shoulders upwards against resistance.*
- *Test sternomastoid function bilaterally by asking the patient to lift his* head off the couch against the resistance of your hand on his* forehead.*

- *Test each sternomastoid muscle by asking the patient to turn his* head in one direction against resistance and observing the strength of contraction of the muscle on the opposite side.*

XII Hypoglossal nerve

The XII nerve is motor to the tongue.

Observe the tongue resting in the floor of the mouth.
  Ask the patient to put out his* tongue and observe any deviation.
  Ask him* to waggle the protruded tongue from side to side.

LMN lesion of the XII nerve will cause wasting and fasciculation (fibrillation) on the affected side of the tongue. When protruded the tongue will deviate towards the affected side being pushed over by the muscle on the intact side.

UMN lesion of the XII nerve will lead to a small tongue with diminished voluntary movements.

The last four cranial nerves are often affected at the same time causing either bulbar (LMN) or pseudo-bulbar (UMN) palsy, particularly in bilateral stroke (CVA) and also in **motor neurone disease**.

6.4   Examination of motor function

When neurological disease is not anticipated, examination of the motor function of the limbs is usually limited to excluding muscle wasting, and testing muscle tone and power around the major joints and the tendon reflexes.

*Note on **inspection**:*

  Wasting or hypertrophy of muscles
  Fasciculation
  Involuntary movements

*Assess muscle **tone** at each major joint in the limbs and document whether it is normal, increased or decreased.*
  *Test **Power** (muscle weakness) of a single muscle or group of muscles supplied by a nerve whose root base is known.*
  Initially, determine whether any abnormality affects a limb or limbs globally (lateralising sign) or a single group of muscles (localising). The degree (grade) of muscle weakness is recorded as follows:

0 *No contraction*
1 *Flicker of contraction*
2 *Active movement with gravity eliminated*
3 *Active movement against gravity*
4 *Active movement against gravity and resistance*
5 *Normal power*

Percussion may be carried out by gently tapping a relaxed muscle with a tendon hammer or finger tip (if reflexes are very brisk) to precipitate fasciculation.

*Elicit **reflexes** by demonstrating superficial (abdominal) and deep (tendon) reflexes. These must be carried out with the patient in as relaxed a position as possible.*

Tendon reflexes are elicited by gently tapping the tendon directly (or with your finger on a tendon) with the head of a patella hammer and observing the appropriate muscle contraction. The hammer should have a full length, flexible (preferably plastic) handle and be held in a position which allows the hammer-head to fall onto the tendon rather than strike it. Practise handling a patella hammer in such a way that it is allowed to fall, and you will find that you are holding it about one third of the way from the end. The tendon should be struck perpendicular to its length with the aim of causing a brief stretch of the muscle which then reflexly contracts. It is important to observe the muscle that is expected to contract and each reflex should be considered in terms of its nerve root base and graded as follows:

Grade	Notation
Normal	$+$
Reduced	$+/-$
Absent	$-$
Increased	$++$

Elicit each reflex once only and make immediate comparison with the same reflex on the opposite side. The reflexes should be symmetrical and it is the difference between the two sides that is important.

If a tendon reflex appears to be absent, test it again with reinforcement (Jendrassik's manoeuvre) which distracts the patient from over-riding the reflex, as follows:

When testing lower limb reflexes ask the patient to lock together the fingers of both hands and try to pull them apart on the command 'pull' and then repeat the reflex.

When testing the upper limb reflexes the patient should be asked to clench his* teeth on command.

Reinforcement of the reflex lasts only approximately a second, so the patient should be asked to relax and the manoeuvre repeated for each attempt to elicit the reflex.

Fasciculation

This term describes the flickering appearance of unco-ordinated contractions of fascicles (muscle bundles) within a muscle. The patient should be warm (because shivering may be confused with fasciculation) and the muscles should be viewed in good light. Percussion with patella hammer or finger tip may precipitate fasciculation. The presence of fasciculation suggests denervation of the muscle usually due to abnormality of the motor neurons in the brainstem or anterior horn of the spinal cord. Fascicular twitching of facial muscles, particularly orbicularis oculi (**myokymia**) is usually of no pathological significance.

Tone

This may be:

- Normal
- Decreased – in LMN and cerebellar lesions
- Increased – in UMN lesions ('clasp knife' spasticity and clonus)
  – or in extrapyramidal lesions ('cogwheel rigidity').

Muscle weakness

This may be due to:

- Myositis when the muscle will be painful and tender
- Myopathy or neuromuscular block (eg myasthenia gravis)
- Lower motor neurone lesion
  The affected muscles are wasted, flaccid, with fasciculation and absent tendon reflexes; plantar response is flexor or absent.
- Upper motor neurone (pyramidal) lesion
  The muscles are not wasted, tone is increased and described as spastic ('clasp knife' type) and the tendon reflexes are exaggerated; the plantar response is extensor. In longstanding UMN lesions (as in stroke) there are trophic changes of the skin which becomes oedema-

tous. The pyramidal distribution of weakness includes the extensors of the arms and flexors of the legs where the tone is most increased in the flexors of the arm and the extensors of the leg.

Tendon reflex

This will be diminished or abolished by a lesion anywhere in the reflex arc. Muscle weakness may render the muscle incapable of responding; the sensory component may be affected in tabes dorsalis; the motor side may be affected in poliomyelitis; and both may be affected in peripheral neuropathy.

The reflex will be exaggerated in an UMN lesion but some people have naturally brisk reflexes particularly if they are anxious. It is the comparison of a reflex that is thought to be abnormal with the reflex that is normal that is important.

Tendon reflexes will be:

- Reduced in LMN lesions and peripheral neuropathy
- Increased in UMN lesions

Reduced or absent tendon reflexes at the ankle are common in the elderly.

1 Examination of the neck and trunk

Test tone by gently rolling the relaxed head from side to side on the pillow. In order for the patient to be relaxed, you may need to distract him* by talking or by asking him* to carry out some other task, such as asking him* to clench his* fist.
Test power of:

- Extensors and flexors of the head by asking the patient to lift his* head from the pillow or push back against the pillow.
- Abdominal muscles by asking the patient to sit up from the supine position with arms folded across the chest. You may need to support his* legs by holding them down onto the bed.

Test abdominal reflexes by gently running an orange stick across the skin at three levels of the abdomen on each side (just below the costal margin, the level of the umbilicus and the iliac fossa) and observing reflex contraction of the underlying muscle. Note the grade of reflex in the four abdominal quadrants.

Abdominal reflexes are likely to be absent in very obese subjects, those with poorly developed abdominal muscles (e.g. women after multiple childbirth and the elderly) and in persons who have had abdominal operations. The reflex is mainly segmental but depends on the integrity of the corticospinal tract, so will be reduced on the side of an UMN lesion. The abdominal reflexes tend to be lost early in multiple sclerosis.

2 Examination of the upper limbs

Inspect *for wasting, fasciculation and involuntary movements.*
Assess **tone** *at wrist and elbow – note whether normal, increased or decreased.*
Test **power** *of muscle group groups as follows:*

	Muscles	Root base	Action/test
Hand	Flexors of fingers	(T1)	Grip hands
	Extensors of fingers	(T1)	Extension of outstretched fingers
	Dorsal interossei	(T1)	Finger abduction
	Abductor pollicis brevis	(T1)	Abduction of thumb
Forearm	Flexors and extensors of wrist	(C8)	Flexion/extension of wrist
	Flexors (biceps)	(C6)	Flexion of elbow
	Extensors	(C7)	Extension of elbow
Upper arm	Deltoid	(C5)	Shoulder abduction
	Triceps	(C7)	Elbow extension

Record the degree of muscle weakness.

Assess **coordination** *by asking the patient to touch repeatedly first his* nose and then your finger placed approximately 60 cm away, using first the tip of one forefinger and then the other (the finger–nose test).*

Coordination of movements is governed by the cerebellum and cannot be assessed adequately in the presence of proximal muscle weakness or loss of position sense.

Test tendon reflexes *noting grade:*

Muscle	Root base
Biceps	C5, 6
Triceps	C6, 7
Supinator	C5, 6
Finger flexion	C7, 8

With the patient lying comfortably ask him* to loosely fold his* arms across his* upper abdomen with his* wrists crossed. The tendon reflexes can be elicited from this position as shown in Fig. 28.

The biceps reflex is elicited by tapping the tendon hammer on the examiner's thumb (for the left) and forefinger (for the right) which are placed over the tendon. Contraction of the biceps muscle and flexion of the elbow are observed but contraction of the tendon can be felt.

When the triceps tendon is tapped it is important to note that the muscle contracts. The movement of extension of the elbow does not usually occur unless the response is brisk.

The supinator jerk may be demonstrated by tapping directly over brachioradialis (where a wrist watch is normally worn), or by striking the examiner's finger or thumb which is placed over the tendon above the wrist, because direct percussion may be painful.

The finger flexor jerk is elicited by tapping the palmar surface of the fingers which are slightly flexed. Hoffman's reflex is performed by passively flexing the terminal phalanx of the index finger of the pronated hand and releasing it with a sharp flick. A positive response to both these reflexes consists of flexion of the fingers and suggests muscular hypertonia or hyper-reflexia.

3 Examination of the lower limbs

Inspect for wasting, fasciculation and involuntary movements
Assess **tone** at hip, knee and ankle.

Clonus may be demonstrated at the ankle by sudden sustained dorsiflexion of the foot. If the response is positive you will feel the foot move rhythmically upwards and downwards at the ankle.

Clonus is associated with an UMN and increase in tone (spasticity).

Test **power** of individual muscles or muscle group and note grade of muscle weakness when present.

	Muscle	Root base	Action
Hip	Flexors	L2,3	Lift up leg
	Extensors	L5, S1	Press leg into bed
	Abductors	L2,3	Press knee outwards
	Adductors	L2, 3	Press knee inwards

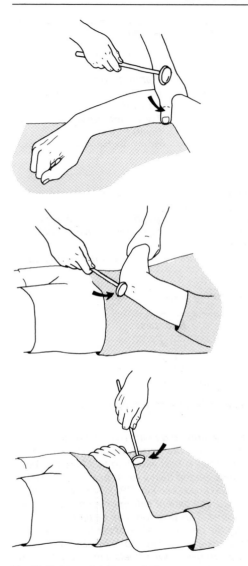

Fig. 28. Reflexes of the upper limb.

	Muscle	Root base	Action
Knee	Flexors	L5, S1	Flexion of knee joint
	Extensors	L3, 4	Straighten knee
Ankle	Flexors	S1, 2	Plantar flexion
	Extensors	L4, 5	Dorsiflex ankle or pull big toe upwards
Foot	Evertors	L5	Twist foot outwards
	Invertors	L5, S1	Invert foot

Assess co-ordination

- Ask the patient to rub his* heel slowly up and down the opposite shin starting at the knee.
- Ask him* to touch your forefinger (held about 10 cm above his* opposite knee) with his* great toe (the equivalent of the finger–nose test for the upper limb).
- Ask the patient to tap his* foot repeatedly against your hand.
- Observe gait.

Test tendon reflexes noting grade:

Reflex	Root base
Knee	L3, 4
Ankle	S1, 2
Plantar	S1

If tendon reflexes appear to be absent, test again with reinforcement.

The knee jerk is elicited by tapping directly over the quadriceps tendon between the patella and the tibial tubercle. The knee must be flexed and relaxed and this is best achieved by lifting the legs (or leg if the patient's legs are too heavy to lift both together) and supporting them under the knee (see Fig. 29a). The reflex may also be demonstrated with the patient sitting on a chair with one knee crossed over the other. This position may be particularly useful in demonstrating the pendular reflex of cerebellar disorder.

Demonstration of the ankle jerk is best done by asking the patient to splay his* legs 'frog-like' with heels almost together. A slight stretch can be given to the Achilles tendon by dorsiflexion of the foot and the tendon struck directly. A positive response is

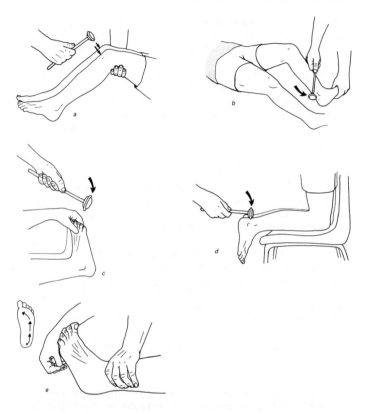

Fig. 29. Reflexes of the lower limb.

plantar flexion at the ankle and this can be seen and felt by the examiner's hand which is holding the foot (see Fig. 29b).

The position described above may be difficult to achieve for elderly patients and those with hip-joint disease. The ankle jerk may then be demonstrated by asking the patient to straighten his* legs with feet vertical. The examiner's hand is placed over the plantar surface of the foot and dorsiflexion achieved by striking the hand with the hammer (see Fig. 29c).

An alternative position involves the patient kneeling on a chair with feet dependent over the edge and the Achilles tendon struck from above (see Fig. 29d).

***Plantar response** (Babinski) is elicited by gently running an orange stick along the outside of the sole of the foot from the heel to the little toe, and coming round towards the big toe (see Fig. 29e).*

Warn the patient in advance of what you are going to do and ask him* to look at the ceiling. Many patients have sensitive soles of their feet so it may be necessary to distract their attention by asking them to talk, or to perform a Jendrassik manoeuvre and to secure the leg from withdrawal by gently holding the ankle.

Plantar flexion of the toes, usually associated with dorsiflexion of the foot at the ankle, is the normal response to the stimulus described above after the first year of life and is termed the flexor response (or Babinski negative). It is a segmental reflex at S1 and when abnormal (extensor or positive) indicates an organic lesion of the corticospinal tract. The positive response is extension of the great toe ('upgoing toe') with fanning of the other toes. With a lesser degree of corticospinal tract damage the response may be flexor but less vigorous than normal but this may still be significant. In addition, the degree of stimulation required to elicit a response will vary so that in severe damage to the corticospinal tract a brisk extensor response may be produced simply by touching the heel of the foot. Thus, there is a spectrum of response depending on the extent of the damage to the higher cerebral centres.

An abnormal response may be observed in deep sleep or coma from any cause (particularly following a seizure) presumably because the corticospinal tract fibres are functionally depressed.

Gait

The patient should be asked to walk away from you, turn and then walk towards you while you observe his* gait. He* should then be asked to walk heel-to-toe in a straight line (tandem walking). It is often helpful to ask the patient to stand with feet slightly apart and arms outstretched, close his* eyes and then stand on tip-toe. Satisfactory performance of this manoeuvre makes it unlikely that there is clinically significant deficit of power or coordination.

*In the **Romberg test** the patient is asked to stand straight with eyes open and feet together. When he* has his* balance, ask him* to close his* eyes. A positive response (i.e. unsteady when eyes are shut but steady with eyes open) suggests loss of position sense in lower limbs. Unsteadiness even when eyes are open suggests a cerebellar cause for ataxia.*

Common disorders of gait include:

- Waddling
  The patient rocks from side to side as he* walks. This is due to proximal myopathy and the diagnosis may be supported clinically by asking the patient to rise from the sitting position without the use of his* arms. He* will find this difficult or impossible because of proximal muscle weakness. Symptoms will include difficulty in climbing the stairs.

- Shuffling
  Small shuffling steps ('*marche à petits pas*') characteristic of Parkinson's syndrome.

- Stiff
  Legs move with a circular motion with the toes tending to scuff the ground. Due to spastic paraparesis.

- Ataxic
  Broad-based gait, unsteady on turning and poor heel–toe walking. Due to cerebellar dysfunction.

- Foot drop
  Initially the affected foot is lifted high off the ground and brought down with a 'slap'. There is then a tendency to scuff the toe of the shoe on the ground as the foot cannot be raised as the leg is advanced and finally walking is only possible by swinging the affected leg in a circular motion to prevent the toe from scraping the ground. Due to common peroneal nerve palsy or L5/S1 root lesion.

- Hemiparetic
  There is circumduction of the affected leg which is extended. The pelvis is tilted upwards on the ipsilateral side. Due to previous stroke.

- Stamping
  The feet are lifted high (to avoid minor obstruction) and are brought down forcefully to the ground. Due to loss of posterior column sensation. This gait is now rarely seen as the commonest cause is tabes dorsalis (neurosyphilis).

6.5 Examination of sensory function

Testing sensory function is often difficult and time consuming and therefore is usually performed in detail only when indicated. The indication may be obvious, as when the patient has sensory symptoms or has a laceration that may have damaged a sensory nerve. Sometimes, however, the sensory system is examined to seek an abnormality of which the patient is unaware (such as peripheral neuropathy in a patient with diabetes).

For the assessment to be meaningful, it is vital that the patient is relaxed, that the examination is not prolonged and that the patient does not see the various stimuli which are to be administered. It is also important that he* is a good sensory witness, and that he* knows before the test what the stimulus is to be, and what is required of him*.

The assessment of sensory witness may be tested if the patient has no abnormality of the auditory nerve by asking him* which ear detects the sound of a tuning fork that is placed vibrating in the middle of the forehead, while the examiner's finger blocks the external auditory meatus of one ear. Inaccurate localisation to the uncovered ear suggests that he* is a poor sensory witness. In these circumstances, it is suggested that the sensory examination should be gross and brief, since a more detailed examination may not yield reliable information. The testing of sensation is entirely subjective and the results should be assessed with this in mind.

When examining sensation note:

1 That appreciation of certain sensory stimuli is reduced or altered and
2 The distribution of the sensory loss

Test the following after explaining to the patient what you are going to do. Begin by asking the patient to close his* eyes so that he* is unaware of the nature of the stimulus and its site:

- *Light touch, using cotton wool stroked gently on the skin.*
- *Superficial pain, using the blunt and then the sharp end of a disposable neurological pin. It is important that the pin be disposable and used on only one patient because of the possibility of transmission of blood borne diseases such as HIV and hepatitis B. The stimulus should not be so sharp that it is painless and it should never draw blood.*

  It is important to establish that the patient can localise the stimulus by identifying where it is applied and can recognise as double two points simultaneously applied to the skin (tactile discrimination). In addition, a stimulus should be applied to both limbs at the same time and the patient asked to determine whether one or both sides are being touched (sensory inattention).
- *Deep pain, by squeezing the Achilles tendon or applying pressure over a terminal phalanx.*

- *Temperature, by comparing the appreciation of hot and cold objects. This is performed formally by using two test tubes one containing hot water and the other cold. A less formal test involves the use of the tuning fork as a cold object.*
- *Position sense, by moving the terminal phalanx of a finger or toe in an upward or downward direction and asking the patient to identify the direction of movement. The phalanx should be held at the two sides so that it is not pressure on the upper or lower surface which is identified. If position sense is lost at the phalanx then move to more proximal joints (ankle and wrist).*
- *Vibration sensation, which is the tingling felt when a vibrating tuning fork is applied to a bony prominence. Start with the great toe or index finger and work proximally using the styloid process, elbow, medial maleolus, tibial tubercle.*
- *Appreciation of form (stereognosis), which is tested by asking the patient to identify a coin (20p or 50p) or a key placed in his* hand or to identify a number or letter 'written' with a pencil on the palm.*
- *Recognition, of familiar objects.*

Characteristic distribution of sensory disturbance helps with diagnosis as follows:

- Peripheral nerves
  The distribution of sensory loss corresponds to the cutaneous area supplied by the nerve affected (see Fig. 30). All modalities of sensation are lost but if the lesion is incomplete there may be tingling (rather than numbness) in the distribution of the affected nerve. In addition, there may be loss of power suggesting a LMN lesion.
  When peripheral nerves are diffusely affected as in **polyneuropathy**, the distribution of sensory loss is 'glove and stocking'. A common cause of peripheral neuropathy is diabetes and an essential part of the assessment of such patients is examination of peripheral nerve function (particularly vibration and pain sensation).
- Spinal nerve root lesion
  The symptoms are referred to the distribution of one or more dermatomes (see Fig. 30). Very often the presenting symptom is pain due to irritation of a nerve root.
  Note that T4 root distribution is at nipple level and T10 corresponds with the umbilicus.
- Spinal cord
  A lesion limited to one half of the spinal cord produces dissociated sensory loss (**Brown-Séquard syndrome**). Impairment of the poster-

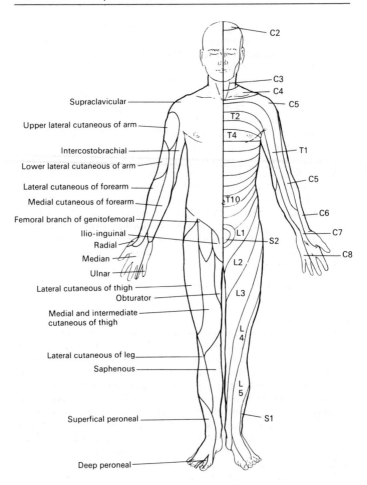

Fig. 30. Dermatomes and peripheral nerves (a) Anterior view.

ior columns causes ipsilateral loss of position sense and vibration, and impairment of the spinothalamic tract causes pain and temperature loss on the contralateral side. Transection of the cord leads to loss of all modalities of sensation below the lesion so that there is a

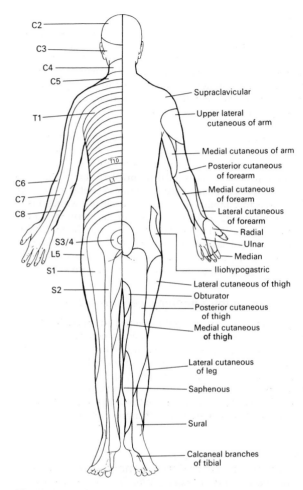

Fig. 30. (continued). (b) Posterior view.

'sensory level' above which sensation is intact. Degeneration of the posterior columns (tabes dorsalis and subacute combined degeneration of the cord due to pernicious anaemia) causes loss of position sense and vibration.

- Sensory cortex
  Cortical sensory loss is manifest by sensory inattention and unilateral neglect, astereognosis, reduced two-point discrimination and reduced ability to localise a stimulus. Agnosia is the inability to recognise objects and is usually further defined as visual, auditory or tactile. Lesions of the non-dominant occipito-parietal region lead to visual agnosia in which the patient is unable to recognise familiar objects that he* clearly sees.
- Hysterical sensory loss
  This is characterised by a distribution of sensory abnormality that corresponds with the patient's idea of the body rather than with anatomical nerve supply. The demarcation between normal and abnormal tends to be very sharp and often involves abrupt change at the mid-line or at the circumference of a limb. A useful test (which can also be used to establish reliability as a sensory witness) is to place a vibrating tuning fork on each side of the sternum in turn. Appreciation of the vibrating sensation depends on bone conduction and not on superficial sensory pathways limited to dermatomes. Thus, one should be suspicious of an hysterical sensory loss if the patient claims that the sensation is different on the two sides.

6.6   Examination of the autonomic nervous system

The autonomic nervous system is not examined routinely but symptoms such as postural hypotension, diarrhoea, impotence and loss of ability to sweat for which no other cause can be found, may suggest autonomic neuropathy. In addition, diabetes may be frequently complicated by autonomic neuropathy which may affect cardiac response to stress (such as surgery) and the testing of patients with diabetes (particularly if the disease has been present for > 10 years, or the ankle reflexes are absent) should be part of the routine examination.

Test by confirming:

- *Increase in heart rate on standing*
- *Variation in heart rate during **Valsalva manoeuvre**. This is forced expiration against a closed glottis but a patient will not normally be able to understand this instruction. Ask him* to pretend that he* is blowing up a balloon or straining at stool. A more reproducible method is to attach a 2 ml or 5 ml syringe barrel to a sphygmomanometer and ask the patient to blow to maintain a pressure of 40 mmHg for 15 s.*

    Record an ECG (any lead which has a good positive R wave)

for a baseline period, during the Valsalva manoeuvre and for at least 30 s afterwards. Measure the minimum R–R interval (usually just after releasing) and the subsequent maximum R–R interval.

During the Valsalva manoeuvre the raised intra-thoracic pressure reduces venous return and blood pressure initially falls. There is then a compensatory tachycardia and blood pressure returns to normal with peripheral vasoconstriction mediated by the sympathetic nervous system. When the pressure is released there is an overshoot of blood pressure and vagally induced bradycardia. The blood pressure responses can only be assessed with continuous intra-arterial measurements so it is variation in heart rate that can be readily recorded which is used routinely.

The ratio of the longest to the shortest R–R interval should exceed 1.4 and autonomic dysfunction is suggested if the ratio is less than 1.1 (fixed R–R interval).

6.7 Minimal statement of the central nervous system (CNS)

Alert, cooperative and orientated in time and place
Right handed
Skull and spine normal
No dysarthria/dysphasia
Pupils equal, regular, react equally to light and accommodation (PERLA)
Optic fundi normal
Eye movements (EOM) full and equal. No nystagmus
Upper limbs – tone, power, coordination sensation normal
Lower limbs – tone, power, co-ordination sensation normal
Tendon reflexes – all present and equal, plantars flexor

7 Examination of the locomotor system

● *Inspect each joint for:*
Swelling
Erythema
Deformity
Muscle wasting

- *Palpate each joint for:*
  Warmth
  Tenderness
  Cause of swelling – fluid, soft tissue, bone
  Range of movement – passive and active
  Instability
  Crepitus

Measure true and apparent shortening of the legs

Joint swelling has three important causes:

Effusion, this is fluid within the joint and may occur in excess in almost any condition (the normal amount of synovial fluid is not clinically detectable). Analysis of aspirated fluid may give valuable diagnostic information.

The fluid nature of the swelling can be determined by noting fluctuation and also the movement of the swelling from one compartment of the joint to another. Fluid in the knee joint can be confirmed by the **patella tap** test. With the leg held straight any fluid in the supra-patellar pouch is squeezed into the main knee compartment with the left hand while the right hand gently pushes the patella posteriorly against the femoral condyles. In the presence of fluid there is a characteristic sensation of the patella tapping against the underlying bone.

Synovial thickening which is characteristic of rheumatoid arthritis.

Bony swelling which is characteristic of osteoarthritis and can be seen frequently in the distal interphalangeal joints of the hands (Heberden's nodes).

Warmth of the skin overlying a joint is assessed by the examiner using the back of his hand to compare the temperature with the joint on the opposite side or with skin not overlying the joint. Warmth and erythema suggest active inflammation, such as gout or bacterial infection (septic arthritis).

The range of **joint movement** is assessed subjectively or objectively using a goniometer, and is expressed as degrees of flexion or extension when compared with the neutral position of the joint. The neutral position of each joint occurs when the patient adopts the 'anatomical position' – i.e. standing to attention with palms pointing forwards. The only exception is the forearm, where the neutral position is with the elbow by the side and flexed at a right angle with thumb pointing upwards.

Deformity is the term used to describe two types of joint abnormality.

1. Where opposing joint surfaces have partly lost contact with each other. This typically occurs in the **subluxation** of the metacarpopha-langeal joints in rheumatoid arthritis.
2. Where the alignment of the joint is altered. When the part distal to the joint is aligned away from the mid-line the term **valgus** deformity is used, and **varus** deformity when displaced towards the mid-line.

A coarse grating which is both heard and felt when a joint is moved (**crepitus**) indicates rough bone surfaces in contact and is typical of osteoarthritis.

Leg shortening

Measure the length of each leg from the anterior superior iliac spine to the medial malleolus (true length).

Measure the distance from the umbilicus to the medial malleolus of each leg when any difference will be due to 'apparent' shortening.

A difference in true length indicates that the shorter leg has disease of the hip joint, or fracture of the femur on that side. If there is apparent shortening it is likely that there is tilting of the pelvis due to adduction deformity of the hip.

VI Documentation of the medical record

1 Documentation of the medical record

The history and examination should be recorded as already described. In addition you should:

1. Summarise the history and examination (positive findings)
2. Construct a provisional or differential diagnosis
3. List investigations required and tick off those requested
4. Decide upon a plan of management
5. Write up progress notes (and operation notes)
6. Write your own discharge note
7. Note the final diagnosis/diagnoses

1. Summary of positive findings

This should include the salient features of both history and examination: e.g. 74-year-old retired plumber with a 24 h history of chest pain and breathlessness. On examination there were features of congestive cardiac failure.

2. Provisional or differential diagnosis (or Problem list, see Problem Orientated Medical Record)

This should be written out in the true sequence of events, thus:

- Aetiology
- Pathological process
- Structural lesion (if any)
- Disorder of function (if any)

For example:

Chronic rheumatic carditis
Mitral stenosis
Atrial fibrillation
Cardiac failure.

3. Special investigations

The results of special investigations should be included in the progress notes and when there is a series of investigations (for example serial blood counts, serum electrolytes, erythrocyte sedimentation rates) the results should be documented on a flow sheet, or as a graph on squared paper. This helps to identify trends and helps to reduce the number of blood tests. Such a flow sheet should be filed at the front of the notes for easy access during the in-patient stay and also in the out-patient department.

4. Plan of management

A clear statement as to the proposed course of action in the management of the patient is very helpful, not only to you, but also to a member of another clinical team who is looking after the patient in your absence. There should be a clear indication if (after discussion) the patient is unsuitable for cardiopulmonary resuscitation (Do Not Resuscitate order).

5. Progress notes

You should write brief notes on your patients every day. Documentation that the clinical condition has not changed may be just as important as recording changes. Record any action that has been taken as a result of positive investigations and also any progress report given to relatives.

If you attended the operation make your own notes, but if not, summarise the official operation notes.

6. Discharge note

A full statement of the patient's condition on discharge should be written (including a list of any medication at the time of discharge) and a note make of his* destination (such as home, convalescent home, other hospital). Recommended after-care should be noted, and an estimate made of the prognosis. It is also important to note what the patient and his* relatives have been told about his* clinical condition, its treatment and prognosis. If the patient dies, you should attend the post-mortem and then complete the notes by a short account of the autopsy findings.

7. Final diagnosis/diagnoses or final problem list

The final diagnosis or diagnoses reached at the time of discharge, or as confirmed by post-mortem, must be given in every case.

2 Problem orientated medical record (POMR)

The Problem Orientated Medical Record (POMR) differs little from the conventional record except that there is greater emphasis on the construction of a complete list of the patient's problems. One of the advantages of this system is that problems and the follow-up of problems are not forgotten. In addition, the information is more readily computerised. This account will simply outline the principles of constructing such records. (For full account see Weed, L.L. Medical records that guide and teach. *New England Journal of Medicine* (1968); **278**, 593 and 652.) Some hospitals use this system rather than the more conventional system illustrated previously, but it is always instructive to attempt to produce a problem list.

The record has four parts:

- Data base
- Problem list
- Initial plans
- Follow-up notes

The **Data base** is the conventional record of the history and examination, and includes investigations. Data collection is a continuing process and information obtained after the initial clerking should be added.

The **Problem list** is a complete list of all the patient's problems (separated into active problems and inactive problems) derived from the data base. Each problem is given a number, its date of entry is recorded and the list is then placed at the front of the notes.

Problems may be:

- Precise diagnoses
- Pathophysiological states, such as cardiac or respiratory failure
- Symptoms, abnormal physical signs, and abnormal investigations that are not encompassed by a disease or syndrome already on the list
- Psychiatric problems

- Social problems
- Risk factors
- Past illnesses

These problems should be statements of fact, not hypotheses, or guesses, and should be stated at the highest level compatible with the facts and your understanding of them. If a patient has abdominal pain and you do not know the cause, then 'abdominal pain' is listed as the problem. However, if you have evidence that the pain is due to duodenal ulcer then 'duodenal ulcer' is the appropriate title.

Initial plans. Having identified and recorded the problems the POMR system then considers each active problem separately under the following headings with a statement about each being recorded where appropriate:

- Goal
  For example the level to which blood pressure is to be lowered.
- Diagnostic information required
  The list of investigations necessary to confirm a diagnosis or assess the prognosis of the condition.
- Monitoring required
  This includes measurements such as temperature, weight and pulse rate or serial laboratory tests.
- Treatment
  This includes all forms of treatment (or management) such as surgical operation, physiotherapy, occupational therapy and diet rather than just treatment with drugs.
- Patient education
  This includes a statement about what the patient and/or a relative is told about his* condition and instruction about practical procedures – e.g. that a patient with diabetes has been taught how to draw up and inject insulin, to care for the syringe and to measure his* own blood glucose concentration.

Follow-up notes are essentially the same as in the conventional system except that the POMR considers each active problem separately under the following headings:

- Subjective information – which means documentation of any change in symptoms.
- Objective information – such as changes in physical signs or the results of investigations.
- Assessment – which means re-assessment of the problem in the light of the above information. This may enable a vague problem

title to be changed to a more precise one, e.g. 'abdominal pain' may be changed to 'duodenal ulcer' and the problem list amended accordingly.

● Plan – which is treated in the same way as 'initial plans'.

3 Case illustration

Mr R. Jones, 1 Florence Way, Cambridge CB3 2RB
DOB: 14.3.36
Hospital number: 67 89 04

19.7.93
1600 h

Age 57, Baker

Admitted as an emergency at the request of Dr A. (general practitioner) to CCU under the care of Dr Z. (admitting consultant).

c/o 1. Chest pains 3/52
    2. Shortness of breath 2/7

HPC

Very fit until 3/52 ago when he began to feel unwell and to suffer episodic retrosternal chest pains which were dull in character with radiation to the throat. Never very severe. Tended to come on after the evening meal and also when travelling to work by bicycle. Duration 15–30 min.

10/7 ago severe episode of chest pain lasting all evening and keeping him awake until the early morning.

Since then one further episode of pain possibly related to exertion but unaffected by posture or breathing and unrelieved by milk or Rennies. Not associated with breathlessness or sweating.

1/52 Mild non-productive cough.
    No wheeze
    No palpitation

2/7 noticed that he could not climb the stairs without stopping for breath. SOB increased since then and now breathless at rest.

Last few days slight ankle swelling.

PMH

General health good

1960 (age 38) Duodenal ulcer confirmed by barium meal; 2/52 IP Whipps Cross Hospital; Trouble for two years but then symptom-free until now

No diabetes, rheumatic fever or tuberculosis

No jaundice

No operations

FH

No diabetes, heart disease or peptic ulceration

F	†78 MI
M	92 a&w
S	55 Hypertension taking medication
B	62 Well

SH

Baker for 30 years – flour dust + +

Smokes 25 cigarettes per day,

Alcohol socially only

Lives with wife and two sons in their own home

No social or financial problems

Allergic to penicillin (developed an urticarial rash and wheeze when given penicillin for a sore throat)

No other allergies

No medication other than Rennies

FE

General health good. Sleeps well.

CVS

As above

RS

As above

AS

Weight steady

Appetite good

No nausea or vomiting
No abdominal pains
No dysphagia, acid regurgitation or heartburn
BOR × 1 Normal stool. No blood

GUS

No dysuria, nocturia or frequency
Good stream
No haematuria

CNS

No headaches
No fits, faints, LOC
Vision normal
Hearing normal
No dizziness
No weaknesses or paraesthesiae
Right handed

Joints

Muscles normal
No back pain

O/E

Looks unwell. Temperature 38.8°C
Overweight
No anaemia, cyanosis, jaundice or clubbing
Not dehydrated
No lymphadenopathy
Thyroid normal

CVS

Pulse 96 per minute, regular
BP (right brachial lying) 140/85
JVP raised 8 cm.
Carotid pulses normal, no bruits
Peripheral oedema to mid-calf
No calf tenderness
No varicose veins

Apex beat – 6ICS AAL normal impulse
No thrills, heaves
HS I + II
S3 +
No murmurs
Peripheral pulses present =

RS

SOB at rest
RR 26/min
Chest shape normal
Movements =
Poor expansion
Trachea central
PN dull at both bases
Bilateral basal, coarse, late inspiratory crackles

AS

No spider naevi
Mouth, tongue, fauces normal
Liver palpable 4 cm
   – smooth and tender
   – upper border normal on percussion
Abd – not distended, soft
   – no masses or tenderness
   – spleen and kidneys not palpable
   – hernial orifices intact
   – genitalia normal
PR deferred

CNS

Alert, cooperative, orientated in time and place
Fundi normal
No obvious neurological deficit but rest of examination deferred
   until patient's condition improves.

Subsequent analysis by POMR system

Data base

As above

Problem list

1. Myocardial infarction   – Restrosternal chest pain
2. Congestive cardiac failure – Shortness of breath
                                – Ankle oedema
                                – Cough
                                – Basal crackles
                                – Enlarged heart
                                – Raised JVP, 3rd HS
                                – Enlarged liver

3. Obesity
4. Pyrexia
5. PH of duodenal ulcer
6. FH of stroke and hypertension
7. Allergy to penicillin
8. Smokes 25/day

Initial investigations

Hb 15.2 g/dl
WBC $12.2 \times 10^9/l$
Urea and electrolytes normal
CXR – enlarged heart, pulmonary oedema with small basal effusions
ECG – recent inferior myocardial infarction

Initial plans

1. Myocardial infarction
Diagnostic information – CK–MB and ECG × 3
2. Congestive cardiac failure
Monitoring   –   4-hourly pulse and BP
                          Examine daily for JVP, pulmonary oedema
                          Fluid input/output chart
                          Urea and electrolytes daily
                          ECG daily
Treatment   –   Bed rest
                          Frusemide 40 mg i.v. stat., thereafter
                          Frusemide 40 mg and Amiloride 5 mg
                          orally od
                          Morphine at night if SOB
Patient education   –   Frightened by shortness of breath
                          Told he has some fluid on his lungs because
                          of heart attack and that this will respond to
                          treatment

3. Obesity

Goal	–	Reach 68 kg within 6 months
Monitoring	–	Weigh 3x/ week in hospital
Treatment	–	1000 calorie diet
Patient education	–	Told of hazards of obesity
		Advised to stick to diet

4. Pyrexia

Probably secondary to AMI but ?chest infection.

Diagnostic information

> blood cultures × 3
> sputum cultures × 3
> CXR
> MSU

? developing DVT Check calves daily

Final problem list

Active	Inactive
1. AMI	
2. CCF	
3. Obesity	
4. Pyrexia – ?DVT, ?chest infection	
5.	DU
6.	FH hypertension
7.	Penicillin allergy
8.	Smokes 25/d
9.	Exposure to flour dust

Appendix I
Guidelines for compiling the medical record

The Medical Record should contain the following:

1. Identification

   The patient's name and hospital number should appear on each page.

   The start of the admission record should contain:

   Name, Hospital Number
   Date of birth
   Address and telephone number
   Next of kin with contact address and telephone number
   Name of general practitioner
   Admitting consultant

   Much of this information will be in the nursing 'Kardex' and patient identification stickers and need not be duplicated.

2. History

   This should be recorded as soon as possible after admission and certainly within 6 h, and before any surgical or interventional procedure. Note the time and date of admission clerking. History should include current medication and allergic responses (which should be included in addition on the treatment card and the front of the case notes).

3. Physical examination

4. Differential diagnosis and/or problem list

5. Plan of management

6. Investigations requested (which should be ticked) or planned, and results received. If frequent investigations are likely they should be entered on a flow sheet so that trends can be easily observed.

7. Further history, clinical examination and assessment by a more senior member of the admitting team, which need not repeat the content of the original clerking.

8. Decision with regard to policy on resuscitation and active treatment.

9. A consent form signed by the patient, or relative, should be included in the case notes where appropriate. Specific, informed consent for invasive diagnostic or therapeutic procedures should be obtained. When consent is not obtained the reason should be recorded in the notes.

10. Observations, continuation and follow-up notes. Progress notes by medical and other professional staff should be recorded as events occur. They should provide a relevant chronological account of the patient's course and may be used to justify clinical decisions.

    Each time a patient is seen a record should be entered in the notes and signed (legibly and so that the author may be identified and contacted – name printed with bleep number). The name (or initials) of the most senior doctor present should appear. Progress notes should be recorded at least every 3 days and more frequently whenever there is a change in management policy or significant clinical event.

    Every visit by the consultant in charge (or a visiting consultant) should be recorded. The consultant should sign the notes if any particularly important clinical decision is made. Visiting consultants will write their opinions in the notes.

    All diagnostic and therapeutic procedures and investigations and their results should be recorded.
11. Information and explanations given to the patient and his* relatives (which may differ) should be clearly recorded.
12. On discharge from hospital the following should be clearly recorded:

    Final diagnosis (diagnoses) using standard nomenclature
    Details of discharge arrangements (transport, district nurse etc.)
    Drugs to be taken home
    Arrangements for follow-up

13. A preliminary discharge note should be completed on the day of discharge and arrangements made for its delivery to the patient's general practitioner as soon as possible. The general practitioner should be telephoned if there is a difficult or urgent problem to be dealt with, and always as soon as possible if a patient dies in hospital.
14. A formal discharge summary should be completed as soon as possible and preferably within 2 weeks of discharge.

It is the responsibility of the hospital to safeguard the information contained in the case notes against loss, damage or use by unauthorised persons. The case notes should be available only to those persons who have responsibility for aspects of the patient's care. It is important that those persons who have access to the confidential content of the case notes do not abuse that confidentiality and that they take every precaution to maintain the security of that information.

Appendix II
Checklist for history and examination

History

c/o
HPC
PMH
FH
Medication and allergy
PH and SH
FE/SR
   Fatigue/malaise
   Sleep disturbance
   Skin rashes
   Joint pain/swelling/stiffness

   SOB
   Chest pain
   Palpitation
   Ankle swelling
   Cough
   Sputum
   Haemoptysis

   Appetite/weight
   Bowels
   Nausea/vomiting
   Abdominal pain
   Dysphagia

   Micturition
   Nocturia
   Prostatic symptoms
   Haematuria
   Menstruation
      Menarche (age at onset)
      Duration of bleeding

Periodicity
Menorrhagia (blood loss), dysmenorrhoea
Menopause, post-menopausal bleeding

Headache
Fits/faints/loss of consciousness/dizziness
Vision
Hearing
Weakness
Numbness/tingling
Anxiety/depression

Examination

General features

Well/ill
Habitus, facies
Temperature
Anaemia, cyanosis, jaundice, clubbing
Other features in hands
Lymphadenopathy
Breasts
Thyroid

Cardiovascular system

Pulse BP (arm, position)
JVP
Carotid pulses
Apex beat, position and character
Precordium – impulses (thrills, heaves)
HS I and II, murmurs, added sounds
Peripheral oedema (sacral/legs)
Peripheral pulses
Fundi

Respiratory system

Shape of chest
Respiratory rate

Trachea, central, deviated
Movements, expansion
PN
TVR
TVF
BS
Added sounds

Alimentary system

Mouth/tongue/fauces/teeth
Abdomen
  Tenderness/guarding/distension/scars
  Liver/kidney/kidney/spleen
  Masses
  Bowel sounds
Hernial orifices
External genitalia
Digital examination of the rectum

Central nervous system

Conscious level
Handedness
Skull
Spine
Dysphasia Dysarthria
Cranial nerves   –   specify fundi (if not documented in CVS)
Upper Limbs   –   Tone
                           Power
                           Coordination
                           Sensation (if appropriate)
Lower Limbs   –   Tone
                           Power
                           Co-ordination
                           Sensation (if appropriate)
Reflexes   –   Tendon reflexes of upper and lower limbs
                           Plantar responses
                           Abdominals

Gait

Locomotor system

Joints if relevant
Skin if relevant

Appendix III
Hints for the approach to a patient in a clinical examination

Introduction

Examiners in clinical medicine at all levels (M.B. finals, Membership of the Royal Colleges of Physicians, etc.) require evidence of facility with basic clinical skills and the ability to interact appropriately with a patient. A good personal 'system' for examination allows you to be sympathetic, caring and considerate of the patient even in the examination situation where, unlike 'real life', the issues at stake are not so much the patient and his* problems, but your success!

A rigid system of history-taking and examination is not advised for form's sake, but a system that you know well and that you have used frequently allows you to apply your clinical skills, while all the time sifting and sorting the information you find, allowing you to plan your next move. This ensures that you miss little and you may benefit from serendipity (unexpected findings) as well as showing consideration for your patient. At all stages in the history and examination it is important to consider a diagnosis or differential diagnosis, and to decide whether a particular finding supports or refutes this.

The method for examining a patient differs little between qualifying examinations and specialist or higher medical examinations, but what is required is a greater degree of style, analysis and accuracy.

The two common areas tested in a clinical examination are:

1 The long case
2 The short cases

The long case

The examiners are interested in your assessment of a patient, particularly with regard to the history, with discussion of differential diagnosis, investigation and management and with your ability to solve clinical problems. You need to be skilled in taking a complete and detailed history, examining the patient and analysing and interpreting your findings within one hour. To be sure of the completeness of your clerking it may be helpful to refer to the check list (see p. 176).

The long case tends to be the easiest part of the clinical examination but it is the only opportunity to demonstrate history taking skills, and clinical problem-solving.

- History

  Always introduce yourself to the patient and enquire how he* is feeling. It is essential that you establish good rapport with the patient as he* will then tend to divulge more information, will be helpful in any subsequent discussion with the examiner and will be able to confirm your communication skills if asked.

  Allow the patient to talk for about 5 min so that you obtain a general idea as to what are the major problems and symptom(s). You can then ask him* specific questions, always considering what you think is the diagnosis or differential diagnosis. It is entirely acceptable to ask the patient what he* thinks is the diagnosis and what investigations he* has had or are planned. You should use this information as a guide and not as a substitute for making your own assessment.

  If the history becomes very involved, you may have to ask the patient more didactic and leading questions. If after a quarter of an hour you are not achieving a comprehensible history, it is better to resort to even more didactic questions which require 'yes' or 'no' answers.

  If you can formulate a diagnosis as you go along, this enables you to ask specific questions with regard to confirmation of the diagnosis and assessment of the impact of the disorder on the patient and his* lifestyle. If you are not able to make a diagnosis, then you will have to continue to 'screen' the body systems in relation to the present and past history and use the data to produce a differential diagnosis.

- Differential diagnosis

  It is useful to make a simple differential diagnosis after taking the history and before starting the physical examination. You may be able to be more direct in your examination, noting negative and positive findings that may confirm or refute items on the diagnostic list. You will then be able to highlight these findings when presenting your patient to the examiners.

- Examination

  Always remember to consider your patient when examining him*; having warm hands and using a warm stethoscope will go a long way to ensuring the best of patient cooperation. If one of the patient's complaints is of pain, take particular care when examining that area and be sure to look at the patient's face to identify any signs of distress.

Remember the 'general' component of the examination. When examining specific systems, you should look for and exclude signs that confirm or refute items on your differential diagnosis and that will have a bearing on the assessment of the severity of the condition and its prognosis. Normal (negative) findings may be as important as abnormal findings. For example, in a patient with mitral stenosis the observation that the heart rhythm is sinus (i.e. normal) is as important as an abnormal finding (i.e. atrial fibrillation). You should continue to gather information while you are performing the physical examination, particularly if an abnormal physical sign is present, which is unexpected from the history.

● Impression/summary

It is very important that you allow at least 10 min after taking the history and performing the physical examination in order to collect your thoughts and prepare for your presentation to the examiners. This time will also enable you to anticipate any questions relating to differential diagnosis, investigations and management and problems to be solved.

You may be asked to summarise your patient's age, occupation, major problems and predominant physical findings and you should be prepared to do this, rather than to recite the whole sequence of the 'clinical clerking'. You should highlight the clinical features relevant to the discussion and these features may be either positive or negative findings from the history and examination.

This exercise is also very useful in clinical practice, since such clinical vignettes ('thumb-nail sketch') are invaluable in, for example, X-ray review sessions, or when other consultant specialists are asked to see your patient.

You may be asked to give a likely diagnosis, or reasonable differential diagnosis, in the light of the history and clinical findings you have elicited. This may be similar to the differential diagnosis you had made after taking the history, but some diagnoses may have been excluded by the clinical examination and unexpected physical findings may have caused you to revise the differential diagnosis.

In preparing a differential diagnosis it is helpful to know that certain common conditions are more prevalent in different age groups. Common conditions occur commonly, and you should not fall into the trap of assuming that patients attending the clinical examination are chosen because they have rare disorders. The appreciation of the prevalence and distribution of common disorders is also important in the out-patient clinic and Accident and Emergency Department as well as in the written examination.

- Investigations

  You should plan your investigations in anticipation of the examiners asking you about them. Investigations may be **General**, which screen your differential diagnosis, e.g. blood count, erythrocyte sedimentation rate, urea and electrolytes; and **Special**, which help to confirm your main diagnosis and which may involve more sophisticated technology and invasive investigations and procedures.

  You should avoid the term 'routine' investigations because no investigation should be carried out if it will not help in confirming or refuting a diagnosis or complication of the prime disease process; or assessing the severity and extent of the condition with a view to determining prognosis and planning management. In general, you should ask yourself 'will the result of this investigation change my management?' In addition, it is important to assess the likely gain in knowledge compared with the degree of risk and discomfort to the patient (the 'cost/benefit ratio').

The short cases

The short case examination tests the candidate's ability and skill in demonstrating physical signs and interpreting their significance in the absence of a full clinical history. This section of the clinical examination has been identified as being the most discriminatory and, therefore, presents the most problems to the examination candidates. It is, however, good practise for establishing the best clinical care of patients.

You will be taken to a patient and asked to examine a system such as the cardiovascular system or an anatomical part such as the leg or the eyes, often after a brief introduction to the patient and his* presenting symptoms. For example, you may be asked to examine the legs after being told that the patient has a 2 month history of difficulty with walking. The system examination should be straightforward, but anything else requires that you should be alert and incorporate information from such bedside clues as, walking aids and diabetic orange squash on the locker, into your examination. However, the clinical skills that you will be asked to demonstrate are those basic ones described in this book, and failure in the examination is usually due to lack of demonstrating adequately these basic clinical skills.

There will usually be a pair of examiners in any clinical examination, one of whom will ask you to demonstrate your skills and the other will observe, although both will be marking your performance. You must listen carefully to what the examiner asks you to do (and do it!) and if there is any doubt about what is required then ask for clarification. It is probably better to do too much than leave out anything, but if for example, you are asked to auscultate the precordium then this is what is required and you should not examine the radial pulse, jugular veins in the neck, etc.

Start by briefly greeting the patient and introducing yourself and then ask him* to get into the optimum position for the examination (for example lying as flat as possible to examine the abdomen). You must be gentle and considerate and always leave the patient covered and comfortable with a word of thanks at the end of your examination. If you have identified an abnormality then proceed to look for other signs that may accompany the one that you have found. However, you must be methodical so that no important sign is missed, but do not waste time. You are likely to be asked to discuss possible diagnoses in front of the patient, so be careful how you do this, and avoid words such as 'cancer' or 'syphilis'.

It cannot be emphasised too much that examiners are observers and will, therefore, detect inexperience, lack of clinical skills, and lack of consideration towards the patient, as much as inaccurate demonstration of clinical signs and their interpretation and poor problem-solving ability. The more practice you have had in clinical clerking and the more you have devised a system that will help you to examine the patient in as considerate a way as possible, the more likely are you to perform well under stress. This applies as much to every day clinical work in managing emergency and casualty admissions and the out-patient clinic as it does to formal examinations.

Examination of the lower limb

This section is concerned with demonstrating how the information in the preceding chapters may be collated, so that clinical examination by disease entity can be built into an examination of any anatomical area or body system using the general examination of the lower limb as an example. This facility is often used in clinical medicine and also forms the basis of the 'short cases' in clinical examinations.

It should be possible, after a general inspection of the limb, to decide

Table A.1 *Systemic examination of the lower limb*

	Dermatology	Cardiovascular		Neurological		Joints		Metabolic
		Arterial	Venous	Nerve	Muscle	Rheumatology	Orthopaedic	
Inspection	Pigmentation Ulcers Infection Purpura Specific lesions	White colour Lack of hair Skin atrophy Nail atrophy	Blue colour Pigmentation Varicose veins Ulceration Lipodermatosclerosis	Abnormal position Wasting muscles Fasciculation Trophic changes Gait	Wasting Hypertrophy Gait	Swelling Position Vasculitis Limited movement	Shape Position Shortening Limited movement Gait	Pes cavus Ulcers Pigmentation Vascular insufficiency
Palpation	Temperature Skin texture Induration Papules Desquamation Oedema	Cold Reduced sensation Pulses +/− or − Capillary return	Warm Pulses + Varicose veins Oedema	Tone Power Coordination Sensation Reflexes	Tone Power Tenderness	Temperature Effusion Mobility	Leg length Mobility	Skin texture
Percussion	NR	NR	NR	Fasciculation Clonus	Fasciculation Myotonia	NR	NR	As CNS
Auscultation	NR	Bruits	Hums	NR	NR	NR	NR	Bruits

NR, Not relevant; CNS, central nervous system.

which body system is predominantly affected and then be able to use the more detailed examination procedure of that single system. It may be that you are unsure, in which case an orderly examination of the following systems will be necessary:

General

Dermatological – infection such as cellulitis
                – immune disorder such as vasculitis

Cardiovascular – arterial
            – venous
            – lymphatic

Neurological – nerve
          – muscle

Joints – rheumatological
      – orthopaedic

Metabolic disorders – diabetes
                 – calcium metabolism
                 – malignant conditions
                 – inborn errors of metabolism
e.g.   haemochromatosis
                        cystinosis
                        homocystinuria

More details of the examination of the above are given in Table A.1.

Index